North Wing And Beyond

The Training of a Medical Student in
the Sixties. . . And What Followed

ANONA PERCY

First published in Great Britain as a softback original in 2019

Copyright © Anona Percy

The moral right of this author has been asserted.

Typeset in Adobe Garamond Pro

Editing, design, typesetting and publishing by UK Book Publishing

www.ukbookpublishing.com

ISBN: 978-1-912183-91-3

For W.D.T.

The author acknowledges the invaluable services of *Miss Alexandra Collinson BA* in preapring this book for publication.

Chapter One

I wanted to be a doctor when I was four years old. That ambition never wavered as I grew. My parents' response to those who enquired about this choice of vocation was tinged with puzzlement.

'We don't know *where* she gets it from.'

I attended a direct grant girls' school, which enabled pupils to sit GCE (General Certificate of Education) O-Levels in Latin and English Literature at the age of fifteen; books studied were Charles Dickens' *Dombey and Son* and *Quentin Durward* by Walter Scott. As one might expect, neither of these volumes endeared the author to teenage girls. Tennyson was the set poet: several stanzas are still embedded in my memory.

In the June of my sixteenth year, O-Levels in Maths, Biology, Physics with Chemistry, English Language, History, Geography and French were sat and passed. These academic hurdles behind us, the class became the Lower Sixth instead of the Fifth Form, and decisions now had to be made about further study – essentially, a choice between the Arts or Sciences. This proved difficult for some of my fellow classmates, but easy for me. Medicine required Biology, Physics and Chemistry. For those pupils studying physics but not Mathematics, a simplified course in Higher Mathematics was available, and included an introduction to Calculus. The latter is still a foreign language to me.

During the Lower Sixth, I began writing to universities and teaching hospitals to acquire a copy of their faculty of Medicine prospectus, and an application form. I was determined to be accepted somewhere, and thus the net was cast wide. London had several teaching hospitals. One application form enquired: 'When did your father graduate from this institution?' My father did not graduate from the teaching hospital in question, nor was he even a doctor: in fact, he had retired from his work with the National Coal Board. London was subsequently removed from my list as a place of study. Instead, I concentrated on the universities which later became the Russell Group, and those in Scotland.

My first interview for entry to read Medicine was in November 1961. I would need to travel to the city concerned the day before my interview, and stay overnight in order to be on time for my 9am start. Arrangements were made for me to sleep in the Warden's Lodging of the Women's Hall of Residence, and I was provided with a map.

I left my local train station on a crisp autumn afternoon, beginning my first venture without my parents. I remember the daylight fading slowly to evening, then to darkness. As the train approached my destination, the scarlet and yellow of furnaces blazed on either side of the track.

Once outside the station, the commercial buildings of the city centre were reached by climbing a hill. Upon this hill stood a stone turreted building, which I discovered to be the town hall. Close by was a broad street, and centrally placed on one side of this thoroughfare was a large provisions store with a restaurant above it, at which I ate a meal, then enquiries were made about buses to take me to the Women's Hall of Residence. The bus conductor agreed to inform me when my transport would arrive at the road on which the Hall was situated. Unfortunately, that particular bus route passed the far end of this road, meaning that I would have to undertake quite a walk through the darkness of a strange city. The stone-built houses on either side of the road were set back in generous gardens. Many had mature trees bordering the pavement, and my feet rustled through piles of golden autumn leaves. Before long, I began to encounter students making their way to the Women's Hall and two adjacent men's halls, traces of their conversations merging and dispersing on the breeze.

Once at the Hall, in the Warden's Lodging, I was allotted a standard single-bedded room with a wash basin and gas fire. There were no matches, but I warmed up once in bed, secure in the knowledge that my alarm clock would wake me up in plenty of time to prepare for my interview and reach my destination.

Interviews were held in the office of the Dean of Medicine. This was part of a Victorian stone-built house on the hillside, which led down to the main university buildings. The Dean was a Scot. I remember only two questions; the first was on tuition fees and how they would be paid, to which I explained my plans for a Scholarship. The next was:

'What will happen if you marry?'

No thought was required. I would simply carry on.

As I was the first pupil to experience a University Interview, I was summoned to the office of the headmistress the following day to relate what had occurred. In her allotted lesson period on Friday morning, she announced:

'Girls, the university was asking Anona about marriage. We need to discuss this subject now.'

There were wry smiles and raised eyebrows around the room as we wondered how she, a 'Miss' S. was going to tackle this subject. Following a brief pause, she instructed us to get out our prayer books – her 'discussion' involved us reading through the marriage service. Those studying biology *did* know the anatomy of the rabbit, but this was the total extent of our knowledge. She eventually swept out of the room after this religious enlightenment, black teaching gown billowing behind her. Our ignorance settled quietly around us.

Other interviews followed with a variety of Deans and Professors. All were an exercise in assessing academic ability and suitability to enter the medical profession. The two, I learnt, are not necessarily combined. Only one interview was unpleasant, not due to the rigor of the questioning, but because all three assessors were chain-smoking. There was a blue fug in the air and each man had a reasonably full ash tray in front of him.

Professor Richard Doll had recently published his work on the association between tobacco smoke, particularly from cigarettes, and lung cancer. I was asked if I thought that measures should be taken to curtail the practice of smoking. Presenting the facts, I discussed various methods for restricting the sale of cigarettes – particularly from vending machines, which could be accessed readily by young people.

'In the end', I concluded diplomatically, peering through the haze at my interviewers, 'it *is* a matter of personal choice'.

My father wanted me to become the school teacher that he had once longed to be, for me to fulfil the aspiration that personal circumstances had prevented him from achieving. I was lectured to on the long course of study for Medicine and the long hours of work once qualified. I also encountered this cryptic comment from both my parents: 'We do not *know* anybody'.

Finally, the only real argument I ever had with my Dad took place. As it progressed, he became more and more subdued, while my forcefulness escalated almost to the point of shouting. I could see defeat emerging in his eyes. Then, very quietly, he said:

'I just can't afford the fees.'

I was exasperated. 'Afford?! Afford?! I'll get a scholarship!'

The Education Committee of my county awarded me a County Major Scholarship, which paid all my tuition fees throughout my course. There was a yearly maintenance grant on which to live, paid in three instalments, one for each term. A separate sum was provided for books and equipment. A thrice yearly travel grant paid the cost of conveying me and my two large trunks to and from the city of my studies. In this way, I trained in the profession of my choice at no expense to my parents.

However, the scholarship came with a proviso. If I gave up my studies for any reason other than academic failure, every penny had to be paid back. My father and I had to sign papers to that effect. In my ignorance, I assumed that every student had a scholarship, and it was years before I realised the costs some parents had to meet – especially if there was more than one child.

Chapter Two

CURRICULUM

1st Year

PHYSICS, CHEMISTRY, BIOLOGY
(For those without these subjects at A-Level)
First M.B, Ch.B Examinations in June

2nd and 3rd Year

ANATOMY, PHYSIOLOGY, BIOCHEMISTRY
Second M.B, Ch.B Examinations in March of third year
  Followed by a term of introductory clinical work. Examinations in September for those who had not achieved the requisite mark in March.

4th Year

PATHOLOGY, BACTERIOLOGY, PHARMACOLOGY
Mornings were spent on hospital wards in groups of eight students, attached to a consultant team.

JUNIOR MEDICINE, JUNIOR SURGERY, JUNIOR PSYCHIATRY
Lectures were held in the afternoons, apart from on Wednesday, which
was reserved for sport or research in the university library.

Part I: Final M.B, Ch.B in June.

5th Year

OBSTETRICS AND GYNAECOLOGY, PAEDIATRICS AND
SPECIALS
Specials included:

Ophthalmology, Public Health, Ear Nose & Throat, Forensic
Medicine, Anaesthetics, Genetics and Dermatology.

Part II: Final M.B, Ch.B in June

6th Year

MEDICINE, SURGERY, PSYCHIATRY
Part III finals in June, leading to Graduation.

From fourth year, the Christmas, Easter and summer breaks were
reduced to a minimum. Prior to this, the Christmas and Easter vacations
were four weeks long. The months of July, August and September were
the Long Vacation.

Once clinical work began, periods of hospital residence and ward
duties continued throughout the year, with attachment to different
clinicians and disciplines. A two-week break in the summer was allowed.

Before the academic year began, all new medical students were summoned to the office of the Dean of Medicine, where they had been interviewed, to register as students of the University. I can still picture the elegant and fearsome faculty secretary, Brenda Severn; she was pale of face, with severely coiffed hair. This was the first occasion upon which we met those with whom we would spend the next five years. Numbers of students reading Medicine had been increased from fifty to eighty per year, and we were the first year of eighty, consisting of fifty men and thirty women. This was a very progressive mix for the early Sixties.

We eyed each other nervously for a while, but some of us summoned the confidence to make introductions. One young Welshman, close to six feet tall with short light brown hair, blue eyes and a snub nose, presented himself as 'Richard Davies from the Rhondda'. He wore a corduroy jacket, a beige shirt with squares outlined in blue, and fawn trousers. He soon struck up a conversation with David Ladds, of similar build with curly brown hair and grey blue eyes. They shared a mutual passion for rugby, as both players and spectators.

Neville Playfair had a long, serious face. Clasping a deerstalker hat, he announced that he was going to become a gynaecologist. That notion was smartly rebuffed by Brenda Severn, who informed the whole room that our ambition was to become Registered Medical Practitioners, and *that* was how the registration form was to be completed.

We were then addressed by the Dean, Dr James McNeil:

'Ladies and Gentlemen,' he began, 'You are entering a period of study which will enable you to qualify to become Registered Medical

Practitioners. From the start of your training, you will therefore conduct yourself in keeping with the behaviour expected of those practising the noble art of Medicine . . . and, it *is* an ART, Ladies and Gentlemen.

Your personal appearance is important to the patient, even if, in the beginning of your training, you have little or no contact with them. You will start off as you mean to go on. It goes without saying that you and your clothing will be clean and tidy at all times. Fingernails will be short and spotless. The hair of the ladies will be controlled, no flowing locks – male hair will be short. Ladies, skirts and stockings are worn at all times; trousers are not acceptable.

Sets of limb bones will soon be distributed for you to study. These belonged to a person, they are not plastic replicas, and they are to be treated with respect, and not be waved around in public. Such behaviour would constitute a breach of the Anatomy Act.

You will rise to your feet when a lecturer enters the room to address you and remain standing until given permission to sit. Members of the Faculty and hospital staff, when you encounter them, will be afforded respect, always. Patients are addressed professionally as Mr, Mrs or Miss. If you forget a name, Sir or Madam is always polite. Standards, Ladies and Gentlemen!'

A few weeks into our first term, we were formally welcomed as students of the University by the Chancellor. Those representing the various Departments that made up the Faculty of Medicine were all in academic dress: brilliant hoods and gowns, with the appropriate academic cap. The formal welcome consisted of announcing the name of the student, who then crossed the dais of the Great Hall of the university to shake the right hand of the Chancellor. He too was resplendent in academic dress, covered in wide gold bands, and a gold encrusted cap embellished with a matching tassel.

There was a minor downside. At the time we entered the university, the Chancellor was a well- known politician who had suffered a stroke, which affected his right hand. Shaking it was comparable to grasping a limp bunch of bananas. Poor man – it cannot have been pleasant for him either.

Chapter Three

The centre of the University was an imposing red brick edifice, constructed around a central courtyard. It was approached by steps that led up from a main bus route in the West of the city. The ground floor on the South side had large cloakrooms for men and women. On the first floor was the Great Hall of the university. Concerts, dinners and guest lectures were held there.

Across the quadrangle was North Wing, a three-storey building containing the non-clinical medical disciplines. The towers between the arms of the quadrangle housed the staircases. As students, we had no access to the ground floor of North Wing, which was devoted to the preparation and storage of bodies for dissection in the Department of Anatomy on the first floor. There was a very good relationship between the Anatomy Department and the city. Every year an open day was held, when those considering leaving their body to the Department could come and see exactly what would happen after death – all went home with the necessary papers to sign, should they decide to go ahead. After death, the body was collected discretely by the Department and the process of preservation began. At the completion of the period of study, the body was released to the family. The cost of the funeral was met by the University. There was no shortage of bodies, and in the summer, medical students from Denmark came to learn, as dissection was illegal there. Bodies were required for both medical and dental students to study. The latter needed a thorough knowledge of the head and neck and some knowledge of the chest and abdomen, but none on the limbs.

The first floor of the Anatomy Department had a lecture theatre on the right of the staircase. On the left were lockers and pegs for outdoor clothing, white coats and briefcases. The dissecting room was across the rear of the building with an offshoot at right angles; there was no door at this intersection, and the dental students were in the offshoot. The dentals tended to be rather rowdy and often had to be admonished about the level of noise.

Early in the academic year, there were twenty dissecting tables in the main room for medical students – four to a body. The first dissecting table in the Dental Students' Laboratory had no body on it, but at one end was a pile of detached limbs that they did not need. Concerned at the levels of noise, one of the Anatomy technicians walked into the Dental Lab, approached the back of a particularly noisy individual and carefully placed a hand on his shoulder. We medics looked on in amusement as his knees buckled and he slowly descended to the floor. The dentals stayed quiet after that.

The designation of medical students to each body was alphabetical, but each four was either all male or all female. When we first entered the laboratory, I doubt any of us had seen a dead body before. The head, hands and feet were protected with gauze dressings under polythene wrappings to keep the tissues fresh. There was a faint smell of disinfectant in the air. Each of us had bought a dissecting handbook from the Student's Bookshop near the Chemistry block and the first area of study was the chest wall. Each student was given a set of upper limb bones and the warning of the Dean was repeated: 'These are NOT to be waved around in public.'

We were required to learn all the anatomical features of each bone, each bump and groove, each muscle origin and insertion, and the dates at which each bone ossified from cartilage. All this knowledge had to be mastered in one week, after which each of us would have an oral examination, or viva, with one of the anatomy demonstrators. The pass mark was fifty, and any failure meant repeating until we passed. The Professor of Anatomy had recently retired, having been joint editor of Gray's Anatomy. In his opinion, nobody could score more than seventy in an Anatomy viva. A score in the upper sixties was remarkable.

Dissection of the body took an academic year of three terms. A viva took place every two weeks or so throughout this period on the area we were dissecting, conducted by the anatomy demonstrators. Following the viva on the bones of the upper limb was another on the brachial plexus of nerves in the armpit two weeks later, succeeded by the branches and relationships of the subclavian artery. We became word perfect on the structures around each organ in the chest and abdomen and the complex folds of the peritoneum. Once we began dissection of the head and neck, the course and branches of the twelve cranial nerves were an examiner's godsend. Much time was expended on the greater superficial petrosal nerve and the posterior inferior cerebellar artery.

We also took an interest in the anatomy demonstrators, some of whom were more helpful than others. All appeared to be in awe of the Reader in Anatomy. Beneath the ubiquitous white coat, each wore a white shirt and restrained tie with matching waistcoat and trousers. Well-polished shoes were de rigeur. Dr R.B was a very helpful demonstrator, quietly spoken with a long pale face and short dark hair. One Monday, the collar of his white coat was standing up instead of lying flat. The Reader had briefly walked into the dissection room and had only seen the back of Dr B., who had gathered a small group together for a tutorial. When one of the more confident individuals amongst us pointed out the position of his collar, he explained:

'There is a reason for that. My wife has been away, and I played rugby on Saturday. My kit was particularly muddy so I decided to do the washing. All my washing fitted into the machine, which I thought would be economical with both detergent and electricity. However. . . .'

He then folded down the collar of his white coat to reveal an almond pink shirt, certainly not acceptable for the time. We were informed that all his 'personal' whites had been dyed the same hue, but he wasn't about to demonstrate this.

There were facilities at the entrance to the dissecting rooms that enabled us to wash our hands before we left. Rubber gloves were only used when dissecting the brain. We arrived one morning to see Dr W. plunging the head of Dr T. under the cold tap, before the Reader caught sight of his flushed face and bloodshot eyes. It had obviously been a very convivial evening, and it seemed that one Welshman was doing the best he could for another from the Valleys.

Throughout our time in the Anatomy Department, Surface Anatomy was taught with the help of an artist's model in her late forties. Each session, she arrived in a turquoise silk embroidered robe, wafting heavy clouds of an Avon perfume called Topaz. The anatomy demonstrators were all male doctors with a few years of hospital experience who had decided to train as surgeons. One in particular showed his acute embarrassment by sweating profusely when he saw the artist's model, constantly mopping his face with a handkerchief.

The first part of the examination process to qualify as a fellow of the Royal College of Surgeons is known as The Primary and is heavily weighted towards anatomy. Teaching and examining medical students was an integral part of the learning process for the demonstrators. It became a battle of wits to try and get a demonstrator onto an anatomical topic that he was inadequately prepared for during a student viva – both individuals benefited from it. Of the standard textbooks, Gray's Anatomy was my favourite. I also bought a half skeleton in a wooden crate from a more senior student. Henry, as I affectionately named him, was one of the best purchases I made in my youth. His skull, to which I made reference throughout my career, was particularly fine; to this day he resides in a box in my loft.

Written examinations in Anatomy, Physiology and Biochemistry were held before Christmas in the first term. The big Anatomy viva was at the beginning of January, and preoccupied our minds over the festive season. This hurdle over, work began on dissection of the chest and then the abdomen, which correlated with the related lectures on physiology, or the function of these organs. The head and neck were a study for the summer term. The brain was studied as a whole and in a series of cross-sectional slices of the preserved specimen. A copious supply of tissues was necessary for these study periods, as each brain had been preserved in a concentrated solution of formaldehyde, the smell of which filled the air and made our eyes run. We were supplied with rubber gloves to avoid pickled fingers.

No new appointment had yet been made to the vacant Chair of Anatomy, and teaching was in the hands of the Reader and the Lecturer. The former was a talented man who excelled at teaching the development of the embryo through a series of chalk drawings on the blackboard. He was artistic in other fields, having submitted a wondrous etching of a dragon on a copper sheet for a University Art Exhibition. I fear, however, that many will remember him with embarrassment due to a certain Medical Dinner.

Each year, the Medical Fraternity held two social functions, Medical Ball in late autumn, and Medical Dinner in late spring. The latter was held in the Great Hall of the university and much thought went into the selection of caterer and guest speaker. One year, it was arranged for a celebrated neurologist with an enviable reputation as an orator to speak, and tickets sold quickly. The Great Hall looked its best for such a formal function; long tables were draped with linen, and there were gilt chairs with rich red upholstery. Elaborate flower arrangements dotted the room. The food was hot, unlike the luke-warm offerings of previous events, and certainly did not disappoint.

With the Loyal Toast and Toast to the University over, the Reader rose to introduce the guest speaker. He spoke well, and captured the attention of the entire room with his prelude. It soon became clear, however, that he was reluctant to stop talking. He went on and on, until at one stage his wife was tugging at the lower end of his dinner jacket as a not-so-subtle hint for him to sit down. After what felt like hours, and to the relief of all, he did so. The guest speaker rose and expressed his thanks for the introduction. His speech lasted around five minutes.

Chapter Four

Physiology involved learning how the various organs of the body functioned, and lectures were followed by laboratory studies with ourselves as guinea pigs. Kidney function involved a twenty-four hour urine collection for each of us, and we were provided with large polythene demijohns. Female students were given a glass funnel to ensure that the voided urine entered the neck of the bottle. It goes without saying that, in order to achieve this, the screw cap had to be undone, or the specimen would be directed onto the floor. However, when one was bursting, and faced with the prospect of a sprint across the quad from North Wing to the ladies' lavatory, this instruction could be forgotten in the quest for relief.

One interesting afternoon was spent getting a small tube from our nose or mouth into the stomach without gagging as it reached the back of the throat. I took myself to a quiet part of the laboratory, where I could stare out of the window at the autumn trees. I decided to avoid the nasal route – too many bacteria there. Quietly, with some gentle effort, I managed to get the tube down on the second attempt. Gastric juice was then collected to assess the acidity of the stomach in a calibration experiment. There had been no lunch for us that day, to ensure a clear specimen. We made up for it later.

Lynne Dye was a very attractive young woman, with blonde hair, sparkling blue eyes and long black lashes. She stood out, not just for her looks, but also for her height. When we were studying the eye and how objects are perceived, small bottles of drugs that have an effect on the pupil were provided for each of us. Each bottle had a cap with a dropper system. One drug was to be selected, and one drop instilled into one eye. Those who chose the Eserine bottle produced a constricted pupil, while homatropine had the opposite effect. Lynne did not read the instructions properly. She used a drop from each bottle, producing one constricted and one dilated pupil and a medical student who was unable to see properly until the effects wore off.

Biochemistry lectures were held in the basement of the Department of Chemistry, down the hill from North Wing in a much more modern building. It took time to walk across the quad, get into our outdoor things and then make our way down the hill and stairs to the lecture theatre. Not infrequently, stragglers were berated by whoever was giving the lecture. One Wednesday afternoon, Richard Davies broke his leg playing rugby, and was encased in plaster of Paris from toes to groin. Crutches were essential for his mobility. For his own safety, he always waited until stairways were clear before carefully descending. There were several flights from Anatomy to the ground floor, then from the cloakroom below the Great Hall to the pavement. He then had to get down the hill to the Chemistry Department, and down a number of flights to the lecture theatre.

The lecturer had already admonished his stragglers, and the lights had been lowered for the start of teaching, when the door creaked open. Richard had finally made it. The lecturer was so angry at this tardiness that he failed to notice the crutches, and embarked on a rather impressive rant. He did not anticipate that the entire lecture theatre would rise to its feet in support of Richard.

It was decided that the medical students would have a Biochemistry practical examination. The afternoon was hot and sunny, and most of the laboratory windows were opened to let out the heat of eighty Bunsen burners. Demonstrators patrolled the room to ensure that there was no collaboration on results, and silence prevailed. I had finished the experiment, and was seated at the bench writing up my findings. Down the middle of each bench was a raised shelf that held glass bottles of common chemical reagents. Over the tops of the stoppers I could see the bent head of Patience Rawlings, who was concentrating on drawing a graph. The temperature of the room fell slightly as a refreshing breeze drifted through the windows on the right.

A short while later, Patience leapt to her feet, shouting, 'Flames! She's in flames!' I stared at her, wondering why she had taken leave of her senses to break the silence of the examination room. Beside me, a demonstrator appeared and quickly turned on the tap at the sink. He manhandled me towards it and thrust my head under the stream of cold water. The refreshing breeze had directed the Bunsen burner flame to the top of my head, and Patience had looked up from her graph to see me sporting a halo of fire. The End of Year Ball fell in the next few days, and that afternoon I had a hair appointment at Bronwen Hughes, much patronised by university staff and students. I asked the hairdresser to do the best she could, and explained that clumps were likely to fall out during shampooing. She managed to disguise the mishap remarkably well, and my appearance was salvaged.

Chapter Five

With our second MB Ch.B exams behind us, we proceeded to our fourth year of training. Lectures took place every afternoon, apart from on Wednesday, and were on Pathology, Bacteriology and Pharmacology: or Pots, Bugs and Drugs. Recognition of particular bacteria and specific disease processes down the microscope illustrated the factual content of the lecture course. In the mornings, we began work in the hospitals of the city, being attached to a consultant for a period of weeks while learning Medicine, Surgery and Psychiatry. At the beginning of each study period, we had to discover which consultant and hospital we would be involved with. Who was in our particular team of students could matter, and some exchanging often occurred. In order to present ourselves, suitably equipped, on the ward at 9am, transport had to be researched. One or two students had cars and were generous with lifts, but knowledge of bus routes and times were studied. One then had to find the way to the correct ward in what was a very large hospital. As a year of eighty students, we were usually in ten teams of eight.

After the blood round, each student was allotted a patient to be clerked by the houseman, who had previously performed the same task to produce the proper clinical record. The initial patient contact may have been made on the blood round, but if not, the bed and the occupant had to be located. Each patient was asked if they agreed to being questioned and examined by a medical student. We knew we had until 11am to complete our task, so there was a certain amount of pressure. At 11am sharp, the consultant ward round began, with the procession around the ward led by the Consultant and Senior and Junior Registrars. The Senior House Officer and House Officer followed behind with the trolley containing all the medical notes for patients on that ward. As students, we were positioned close to the trolley, and usually at the end of the patient's bed. Sister, or Staff nurse, was at the opposite side of the bed to the medical staff with the nursing notes trolley. The other nurses were silent at the end of the ward. All patients were in their beds.

The consultant spoke to each of his patients in turn and listened to the clinical findings and an abbreviated case history. At this point, we were often taught about a symptom, clinical sign or the treatment, that the patient was receiving. We were anxious throughout this period, very conscious of the need to make a good impression and not be disgraced by our ignorance. Nerves could result in a student blurting out a totally inappropriate response. Mary Duckworth was prone to such episodes. In one situation, the patient had been admitted as an emergency, vomiting blood from a duodenal ulcer.

'Now, Miss Duckworth, what do we, as doctors, need to do for this patient?'

The correct answer was to replace the blood lost by suitably cross-matched blood. In the meantime, take a sample for cross-matching and set up an intravenous drip with a saline solution. Poor Mary was too nervous, and suggested the exact opposite:

'Put him on anticoagulants'— i.e, prevent the blood from clotting. We all cringed.

Some clinical teaching was done well away from the patient's bed so as not to be overheard. A male patient had been admitted for investigation, and possible treatment, of a lump in his abdomen. The consultant had demonstrated the lump while curtains were drawn around the bed for privacy. They were now drawn back and we were all at the bottom of the ward out of earshot. The consultant gave a reprise of the clinical history and examination. Malcolm, from our group, was asked to give possible causes for the lump. He began with an exceedingly rare muscle tumour in the abdominal wall. A look of irritation crossed the consultant's face.

'Laddie, let me advise you. Common things occur commonly. Never begin your answer with rocking horse manure. Always start with the most likely.'

When we eight were together at lunch, we asked Malcolm why on earth he had given that answer. 'Well,' he replied, 'I decided to start at the outside and work my way in.'

Logic, of a sort.

Chapter Six

When we began our clinical studies, there was no sterile disposable plastic equipment. Syringes of all sizes were glass. After use, they were rinsed and returned to Central Sterile Supplies for heat sterilisation before reuse. Each syringe was supplied in a sterile metal container, with one end sealed by corrugated metal foil. Around each tube was a beige adhesive strip, which bore an emblem demonstrating that the heat sterilisation process had been completed. Prior to adequate processing, the insignia was invisible. Steel needles were flushed through after use and sent for resharpening before being processed and sterilised in a similar way. As students, we learned which of the sterile glass screw capped bottles to use for the various laboratory tests to be performed on patient samples. There were three different containers for blood destined for three separate departments.

1. Haematology: Blood disease
2. Biochemistry: Analysis of chemicals in the fluid part of the blood.
3. Blood transfusion: For grouping and cross-matching.

Irrespective of the test required, each tube had to carry the unique identification of the patient: their name, date of birth, hospital number, ward and name of consultant. This information was written on an adhesive label around the specimen bottle. The latter was accompanied by a request form duplicating the information on the bottle and giving a brief account of the clinical history, probable diagnosis and investigation requested. This form could not be signed by a student, only by a registered medical practitioner – usually the houseman.

A batch of request forms was on every ward early in the morning for the blood round. We began our clinical work each day by helping the houseman draw off the necessary specimens. Sputum, urine and stool samples were the responsibilities of the nursing staff, but all documentation was still that of the medical staff. Specialised samples of pus or fluid from the spinal canal were accompanied by a request form, which was completed by the doctor who had recovered the sample from the patient. Every sample went into a glass screw-capped sterile bottle with a patient identity label.

All syringes, needles and specimen bottles were kept in a series of pigeon holes in the ward Prep Room. Also stored there were the glass bottles containing liquids for intravenous transfusion. Each bottle was sealed by a rubber bung about 2cm thick, which bore on the visible surface two ports marked with a raised X for the entry of the glass giving tube and glass air entry tube. There was a peripheral steel screw cap for the glass bottle. The bottle was inserted into a steel cage which hung from a hook on the drip stand. The glass tubes to be inserted through the rubber bung had oblique shaped ends, for ease of insertion. The tube of the giving set was rubber and flow was controlled by a steel regulator. Each bottle was clearly marked with the nature of the contents by an adhesive label. At each bottle change, contents had to be checked with the requirement of the patient and that person's identity.

When on clinical attachment, a white coat was essential. These could be found in the ward laundry room. It was rare to locate one in the correct size. Valuables were placed in one pocket and a name badge was pinned to the lapel or breast pocket, which also contained a selection of pens and a pen torch. Suitably equipped, we then entered the ward and chose a batch of request forms for which we, as individuals, would be responsible for obtaining the blood required. The correct bottle then had to be located in the Prep Room and the identity label around it completed. Some questioning might be necessary before finding the patient when specimen bottle, syringe, needle and request forms had been assembled. To achieve the necessary specimen at the first attempt, one had to hope that the patient selected had decent veins.

In the hospital, each ward had a prep and laundry room. A sluice was devoted to the urine bottle and bedpan. The contents of both were inspected, and samples were taken if necessary; the contents were then disposed of and the receptacles were disinfected for reuse. No disposable equipment was used. The cold steel bed pan inhibited many a colon.

Every ward had a kitchen to provide hot drinks and simple food for patients. Meals were delivered from the central kitchen in a heated trolley, but the ward kitchen could provide tea, toast and a boiled egg. This was much appreciated by any patent who had been starved for a diagnostic procedure and missed a mealtime. For the post-operative patient who had been prevented from eating, nothing could beat freshly prepared scrambled egg from the ward kitchen, spooned into the mouth by a nurse.

Sister's office consisted of a large desk at which the Ward Sister worked. Close by was a metal trolley in which the nursing records of each patient were stored. There was also a day book containing nursing observations on each patient. Fastened to the wall was a locked cupboard containing the Dangerous Drugs of Addiction (DDA's): heroin, morphine and pethidine. Various quantities of the drug were contained in glass ampoules. In a locked drawer of Sister's desk was the DDA register which recorded each drug administration with the name of the patient, prescribing doctor, the dose of the drug, who administered it and who witnessed it. There was also a record of the number of remaining ampoules. Administering one of these drugs was therefore an exercise that involved both the medical and nursing professions.

The doctor's office contained the metal trolley holding all the notes for patients. Each set of notes was suspended in a V-shaped division from the sides of the trolley with the name of the patient clearly visible. A desk and chair were provided for the houseman and additional chairs for relatives to be interviewed and students to be taught. Clinical notes were kept up to date religiously. Each ward had at least two side rooms with washbasins close to Sister's office. They were usually used for very ill or dying patients, who could receive attention without the whole ward being disturbed. Very occasionally, a private patient occupied a side room, and they were also used for infectious patients, at that time usually for those with suspected TB.

Two maids, under the authority of Sister, cleaned each ward. Ward Sisters were sticklers for hygiene and had impressive, and inflexible, cleaning regimes; the odour of disinfectant pervaded the entire hospital, even in the administrative offices. The wards were of the Nightingale design, a rectangle with a high ceiling. Tall windows were set high in the wall to let in light but allow privacy. Many wards were tiled to shoulder height or above. The floors were polished wood and beds had to be aligned with a particular floorboard, or line of parquet. Bed covers had hospital corners, and when there was a heavy demand for beds, extra would be brought down from neighbouring institutions and placed down the middle of the ward. The aim was to have some empty beds for when the team went on emergency reception. Some patients were discharged, and others who were not well enough for that went to an associated convalescent home for food, rest and gentle exercise under nursing care until they were fit enough to return home. The system worked.

HOSPITAL STAFF

House Officer

A doctor with a basic medical qualification in medicine and surgery. Each post was for six months and was resident in the hospital with one evening off per week. In the first year after graduation, doctors had Provisional Registration with the General Medical Council. Completion of two six-month posts, one in a medical discipline and one in a surgical discipline, led to Full Registration with the General Medical Council. Thereafter, a yearly fee was payable to maintain registration. Competition for certain house jobs was intense.

Senior House Officer

These posts could be in any medical discipline and were for one year. The SHO was expected to be available to the house officer when required. Most SHOs were studying for a further medical qualification, the Membership of the Royal College of Physicians (MRCP) or the Fellowship of the Royal College of Surgeons (FRCS). Each examination had two parts, Primary and Final. The aim was to pass the Primary as soon as possible. There were also Diploma examinations in Child Health, Ophthalmology, Obstetrics and Anaesthetics. Some posts had a good record for candidates achieving success as there was good teaching and plenty of time for study.

Junior Registrar

Those who were applying for the above posts had usually already passed the Primary in Medicine or Surgery. A variety of junior registrar posts was required to broaden experience of the discipline. Those studying for the MRCP could take posts in Renal Medicine, Haematology, Cardiology, Rheumatology or Respiratory Medicine. In Surgery, there were posts in Orthopaedics, Neurosurgery, Plastic Surgery, Cardiothoracic and Urology. There was plenty to choose from. All posts were competitive, and the advertisement sections at the back of the British Medical Journal and The Lancet were eagerly scanned. No one wanted a gap between jobs. The final examination leading to MRCP or FRCS was the goal at this stage.

Senior Registrar

These individuals were accumulating experience in preparation for a consultant post. Again, many branches of the subject would be covered to obtain the broadest possible experience. This particularly applied to surgery and the emergency cases were usually operated on by the senior registrar. As students, we were in awe of them. All senior registrar posts were open to competition and the performance of the applicant at interview was diligently appraised. Vacancies at consultant level arose by three processes: death, retirement, and, rarely, the establishment of a new post. Senior registrars could be waiting for a long time.

Chapter Seven

During our clinical attachment, we lived either in, or adjacent to, the hospital when our consultant team was on 'emergency take'. This gave us the experience of witnessing patients admitted as an emergency between 5pm and 9am. It was invaluable learning, and it introduced us to those procedures necessary to make the diagnosis or rectify the problem. One of those procedures was the lumbar puncture to retrieve fluid from the spinal canal to diagnose meningitis or haemorrhage. Surgical patients were followed to the operating theatre, and it was here that we learned what a living abdomen looked like – as opposed to the abdomen of the corpse that we had dissected in Anatomy. Surgery during the night differs from surgery during the day for a variety of reasons.

Routine surgery is scheduled for a specific theatre, surgeon and anaesthetist. The emergency case will have a designated surgeon, usually the senior registrar, on take, but a theatre and an anaesthetist need to be found. At night, there is competition for theatre space between General Surgery, Orthopaedics and Maternity, and in a large hospital, other specialised disciplines such as Neurosurgery, Ophthalmology and ENT.

The number of anaesthetists available will depend on the size of the hospital. Some surgical procedures will require specialised nursing staff to be called in from home. This all takes time and the establishment of an order of priority between the various surgical disciplines.

As students in residence, we were shown how to scrub up and correctly don an operating gown and rubber gloves. Once the patient was stabilised, teaching was given by the surgeon when the crisis was over. The anaesthetist would also teach on the type of anaesthetic machine and the gases chosen. As well as maintenance of the vital functions of the patient, they were responsible for any intravenous infusion; during the night, this infusion was frequently of blood.

The level of blood in the glass bottle mounted on the drip stand was falling as the transfusion progressed and the anaesthetist asked two of us to fetch another bottle from the anaesthetic room. We were then shown how to check the information on the bottle with patient details in the clinical notes: name, hospital number, date of birth, consultant, ward. We also had to ensure that the blood group was compatible. The new bottle could replace the almost-empty one. The regulator controlling the rubber tubing of the drip was closed tightly, and the glass tubes of the giving set removed from the rubber bung of the empty bottle.

The two of us were asked to insert these tubes into the fresh bottle of blood. I would hold the bottle steady, while Mary Duckworth would get the glass tubes of the giving set and air entry through the ports marked with an X in the cleaned rubber bung. Such was Mary's determination and anxiety over her part in the procedure that instead of getting the tubes through the ports, she managed to forcibly push the entire bung down into the blood. A red geyser erupted from the bottle, and descended as scarlet rain over us all. The surgeon was least bespattered, but the assistant surgeon, theatre sister and we two students were anointed. The anaesthetist dealt with the next bottle himself.

There are very ill and injured patients for whom regular observation and recording of vital signs is required, usually every fifteen minutes. Pulse, blood pressure and level of consciousness were the most frequent assessments to be made and entered onto the patient charts. As medical students attached to clinical firms, we were a useful source of man power, and gained a lot of experience through helping with these checks.

On one of my Junior Surgical attachments I was asked to 'special' a head injury case through the night. The ward was in darkness, with only one lamp shining in the centre for the night nurse. I was on a chair at the bedside of the patient with the blood pressure monitor on a side table. My pen torch was in the breast pocket of my white coat with my ball-point pens. As my wristwatch had no second hand, I had purchased a stopwatch for assessing pulse rates. During the early hours, I needed to visit the staff lavatory. On my return, although it seemed that nobody had moved, the stopwatch had vanished. I learned a valuable lesson that night: never leave any personal possessions unattended in a hospital.

As students, we did not encounter the relatives of patients. Visiting times were in the afternoon when we were in lectures, and in the evening, when we were at supper if we were in residence in the hospital. The exception was when we were required to special a patient at the weekend over a visiting time.

The patient had been admitted to a medical ward having taken an overdose. Her stomach had been emptied of its contents, but she was still deeply unconscious, and curtains were drawn around the bed for privacy. I had been at my task for three hours and could hear visitors arriving on the ward. The bed curtains were suddenly flung open, and I found myself looking into the face of a very angry middle-aged woman.

'Right. I blame you for this, I blame you entirely. She was not well enough to be discharged, not well enough at all – and look what has happened. She could not cope with her condition and should never have been sent home. YOU are at fault.'

I tried to extricate myself as best I could.

'Madam, I am a medical student performing necessary observations on this patient. I cannot leave her to take you to someone who can address your problem. Please have a word with Sister or Staff Nurse, who will get one of the medical staff to speak to you.'

The patient had a long history of Crohn's Disease, an inflammatory small bowel condition which had led to severe weight loss. For this she had undergone a prolonged period of inpatient treatment; according to her visitor, this had not been long enough.

It was occasionally possible to follow a patient from Outpatient Clinic to ward and then to Outpatient Clinic once again – this was more likely with a surgical problem.

Mrs G had a long history of Ulcerative Colitis, an inflammatory large bowel condition. It had curtailed her life so much that she was virtually housebound and needed the security of a readily available lavatory. The consultant surgeon talked quietly to her about removing the whole of her colon, pointing out that she would need to wear a device to collect waste from her small bowel when the surgery was complete. He informed her of the risks involved in the procedure. She looked at him calmly.

'I have no life now. I might as well be in an enclosed order of nuns. I cannot visit friends, nor the hairdresser or dentist, or even go to church!' Her mind was made up – no risk outweighed the hope of a better existence. Many staff were involved in her care immediately after her operation, and I was amongst them.

Six weeks later, her name was on the list of outpatient appointments for late morning. We heard her name called but it took a while to recognise the person who entered the room. She was beautifully coiffed and beaming, dressed in an elegant tea dress and court shoes.

'I am living again,' she declared. 'I can visit friends and go to church. When I am a little stronger I can even consider going on holiday, because there is no need to be ten feet from a lavatory. Concerts, the theatre . . . I can do it all again.' She thanked the consultant and shook his hand, very grateful for the outcome that had been achieved.

Chapter Eight

The Faculty of Medicine had a very strong Department of Psychiatry. The chair was occupied by a man born in Austria and with a strong overtone of his native language, Professor S. We received him with great expectation, as his reputation as an expert had preceded him. During a lecture, the theatre grew restless. Students were glancing at their neighbours; his teaching was unintelligible. A brave soul raised his hand.

'Professor, we do not understand the concept you are discussing.'

Professor S's eyebrows shot up in indignation.

'MOOTHS. I am talking about MOOTHS. You all KNOW this term!'

We stared at one another, and one by one, admitted that we had no idea what a 'mooth' was.

'Yes, you do! You are just being rude!' he bellowed.

We protested our ignorance, and he became exasperated.

'I will write it on the blackboard!'

Then we did realise what he referred to. The word was myths.

Child Psychiatry was the province of Dr W., a rather austere individual with very decided opinions on the raising of children. According to him, no child was ever to be corrected verbally for bad behaviour or restrained in any way, because such action could do untold damage to the developing personality. I listened to this with interest, because I was aware of a three-child family raised along similar lines. The result had been that any visitor seated on a sofa would experience two children tumbling over the top, and at birthday parties there was inevitably a tussle at the tea table – usually accompanied by a mess that descended onto the carpet, and an array of minor injuries. I related this information to Dr W. when he asked for questions, stating that children must be given boundaries for acceptable behaviour. His response, by any standards, was relatively chilling:

'Young lady, you are advocating a system of control. I strongly suspect that, in the future, you will be found to be a baby batterer.'

The students' residence at one of the city hospitals was known as 'Bedside Manor'. Those students on clinical attachment ate breakfast and lunch there, and there were bedrooms on the third floor in which they slept. For a time, the Warden in charge was a psychiatrist, and one Monday evening he asked to speak to the student firm on take for Medicine. Eight of us gathered round.

'I have been appallingly stupid at the weekend. I want all of you to know what happened, so that none of you repeat such irresponsible behaviour.'

He and a fellow psychiatrist had decided to conduct an experiment on the effects of LSD, then a very new drug. The Warden planned to take the substance, while his colleague monitored its effects on both his body and his mind. What resulted was an extremely bad trip with terrifying hallucinations. Both men knew how long the drug was likely to be active. Unfortunately, the time for normal mental activity to

40

resume came and went, and the hallucinations persisted. It must have been a very potent batch. It certainly taught two psychiatrists, and eight medical students, a timely lesson.

Years later, one of these men was struck off the Medical Register for drugs offences.

Chapter Nine

A s part of our training in Medicine we were introduced to the speciality of Neurology. Apart from the three medical wards at the city hospitals, there was also a specialist Neurology unit in one of the more salubrious outskirts of the city known as the Annexe. From my flat, it was a pleasant spring-time walk up the hill to the top, and then a stroll down the ridge to the large roundabout in the valley where one turned left into a large city park. These parks were very well maintained, and ducks and swans dotted the surface of a large lake. Having walked the length of the park, one crossed a road and entered a second park through which the path began to climb. The Annexe was a brick-built structure set facing east on the slope of a further hill. It had a Plastic Surgery unit as well as Neurology.

As we were just beginning our clinical studies, we were allowed to work in pairs. There is a great deal to remember in taking a thorough medical history so that all necessary information is elicited from the patient. Much needs to be assessed in clinical examination, but particularly in neurology. We were assigned a very pleasant lady with brown curly hair and dark eyes, wearing a silky floral robe. Towards the end of a very detailed history, Mrs C. mentioned that her daughter was a medical student. We realised with horror that she was the mother of one of our colleagues. We both felt that a breach of privacy had occurred, and so decided to speak to the hospital staff; we considered that proceeding to a clinical examination would be inappropriate and perhaps unethical.

'Has Mrs C. made a complaint?'

None had arisen, and we were therefore instructed to carry on.

Dr B., the consultant neurologist, arrived at 11am, and each pair of students related the history and examination findings on their allotted patients. When our turn came, we gave the history that we had elicited, and then confessed that we had been unable to demonstrate any abnormality whatsoever. Dr B. reacted immediately.

'You have not been thorough enough! Did you perform a full examination for sensation?'

'Yes, we tested for perception of pinprick, two-point discrimination, joint position sense and vibration.'

He smiled. 'You may have done; but it was not good enough. Really, as sixth year students, you must perform to a better standard than this!'

The whole group declared that we were not sixth years, but fourth years just beginning our clinical work.

'In that case, there is time for redemption. Mrs C. has only one neurological sign and it is on her left hand. If you had tested her fingers thoroughly, you would have found an abnormality in sensation in the tip of her ring finger, and also in the tip of her little finger. She has lost the ability to identify touch between one point and two. This is the only clinical sign of the brain tumour.' – which was subsequently confirmed.

From our knowledge of anatomy, we could identify the region of the brain tumour. Mrs C. died before her daughter graduated. We learned the painstaking nature of a neurological examination.

The other city neurologist was Dr. C., an older man with white hair who often wore a black jacket with pinstripe trousers, with an immaculate shirt and tie. We had all heard rumours about him.

The young female patient had naturally curly dark hair and a fresh, rosy complexion. She was not unlike Walt Disney's depiction of Snow White. She had given Dr. C. and us, as attending students, a clinical history, and needed to be examined. All her clothing had been removed under a covering sheet. When the examination was complete, the patient made several attempts to raise the sheet up above her waist, but each was deftly prevented by Dr C. Her embarrassment, and ours, filled the room – but Dr. C. was serene. I can still see the face of that young woman after all these years.

Psychiatry and Neurology sometimes overlapped. Mr X. was a pleasant and intelligent middle-aged bachelor who lived with his sister in the family home they had known since childhood. He suffered from a delusion that he would harm his sister, and he was very agitated about it. No physical abnormality could be found on examination, and apart from this delusion, his mental function was normal. In time, with inpatient treatment and medication, he was considered fit enough to return home.

Sometime afterwards, we heard on the grapevine that he had murdered his sister, and then committed suicide. His autopsy revealed a totally unsuspected abscess in one of the temporal lobes of the brain.

Pathology, the study of disease in the organs and tissues, was taught by lecture and through the demonstration of diseased organ specimens in glass jars. We had to be able to identify the appearance of tuberculosis, cancer and inflammatory disease in all body systems. Laboratory sessions were held, in which we sat at microscopes learning how to differentiate different disease processes. There was also a one-week practical pathology attachment, and as part of it we were expected to perform at least one autopsy. Usually, the cadaver was opened by one of the post-mortem technicians, with a long incision from the top of the breast bone to the bottom of the abdomen. The chest was opened with rib cutters, resembling loppers used for pruning shrubs and trees. The skull required an electrically-driven saw. It amused the post-mortem technicians to deny medical students the rib-cutters, and we often had to get through the cartilage either side of the breast bone with a large knife.

The Pathology attachment began at 9am on Monday morning and coincided, for me, with a streaming cold. Absence would not be excused, but there was one advantage: I could not smell anything.

Once the identity of each student had been ascertained, I was taken to one side and given the following advice:

'Go and stand over there with your box of paper handkerchiefs. If there is anything you need to ask, just sing out.'

I was still blowing my nose on Friday morning, and I never did get to perform an autopsy.

Along with the hospital department, the city also had a small forensic pathology room used by the Home Office Pathologist, an ebullient individual from the North-East of England. His domain was tucked away amongst laurel shrubbery. A Coroner's case arose during our Pathology attachment and we were dispatched to the forensic autopsy room. The deceased had been discovered in one of the city parks, hidden in bushes, and had probably been there for weeks or months. Before the body was removed from the refrigerator, the two technicians were instructed by the H.O pathologist to 'get the sprays, and start spraying.' Aerosol cans of air freshener were produced, and the spraying began at the head and foot of the autopsy table.

'Right, get him out now,'

The corpse was placed on the table.

'I will do everything . . . just keep spraying.'

I think four cans of air freshener were used during that session. I was lucky – my nose admitted very little at all.

Chapter Ten

The major disciplines in our fifth year of study were Obstetrics, Gynaecology and Paediatrics. As before, we were in teams of eight students for periods of residence when on call. The city had three maternity units, one central in the city, one north and one in a leafy suburb. I was never attached to the latter but experienced periods of residence at the other two. Every fifth-year student had to perform twenty normal deliveries and witness six complicated births. Each had to be written up in a record book. Afternoon lectures proceeded as normal while in residence. The first maternity residence was at the northern unit. Female medical students on call were accommodated in the Nurses' Home. Setting out at night for a delivery involved contacting Night Superintendent to unlock the door of the Nurses' Home and sprinting across the grounds to the Delivery Suite, hoping that one was on time. It was one of the midwives who pointed out that there was a more efficient way of arranging matters when a female student was top of the list for the next delivery. There was invariably a vacant bed somewhere on the antenatal suite that a female student could occupy. Once the expected delivery was over, the student would telephone Night Superintendent for the door of the Nurses' Home to be unlocked, so she could return to her allotted bedroom for that week. Only one disturbance for Night Superintendent, to get back in – not two to get out and then in again.

Vigilance on the part of the student was required. I was asleep in a cubicle on the Antenatal Ward awaiting a delivery when I was awoken with the words:

'Mrs Y., it is time to take your medication.'

I had no idea what I was being offered, and it took some time to convince the midwife that, as a student awaiting the next delivery, there was no way I was going to swallow it.

It was on this attachment that I was profoundly grateful for the men in my group. A very senior nurse settled her eye on me in a way that gave me shivers. She had short white hair, cropped in a masculine style under a sister's cap. She strode around the hospital and associated grounds enveloped in a cape of forest-green wool, lined with scarlet. When we moved around the hospital as a group, my male colleagues kindly formed a circle around me. I found her sinister, and was totally uninterested in her advances.

In the Sixties, pregnant women with high blood pressure were admitted for bed rest and a salt-free diet in an attempt to get them to full term and a live birth. No suitable drugs were available.

Bed rest was no problem for the ladies, but, as the days passed, many of them developed a craving for salt. Porters or maids were bribed to bring banned items of food to the antenatal wards. Potato crisps with the small blue ultramarine packet of salt were especially prized, and the whole ward might have contributed to the cost of smuggling in a jar of Marmite.

The patient was in her early thirties, and had reached the sixth month of her pregnancy, or twenty-four weeks. She was in a large single room and confined to bed because of the risk of a premature labour. I was the medical student allotted to take her clinical history, when she suddenly exclaimed:

'Something is happening!'

Down went the bed clothes and up came the hospital gown. I could see the upper third of the foetal head. This had to be controlled – it could not be allowed to shoot out and rapidly expand. This was going to be a bare hand delivery and those hands had not even been scrubbed. The emergency call button was on the far side of the room, where neither of us could reach it. All we could do to summon help was yell, and in time we were heard.

That premature baby was anatomically perfect, at least externally, and today it may well have survived. But those were very different times.

Assessing the position of the foetus within the mother was a skill we had to acquire. I was assigned to examine Mrs L. and was dispatched to her room. It was her first baby and the position of the foetal back was easy to determine. Tucked under her ribs was a firm rounded shape, consistent with a head – this baby was in the breech position. Mr A., the Senior Registrar, entered the room to hear my findings.

'Breech presentation, back on the left.'

'Good. Are there any further observations that you wish to make?'

'This is a good size baby.'

'Oh, I don't think so.' He replied, and with that, we thanked Mrs L and left the room.

Once out of earshot I was severely reprimanded for my remark about the size of the baby.

'Of course, it is a big baby, but we do not make that kind of comment in front of the patient. After all, she is the one who has to push it out.'

As the foetus was breech, I had concerns that the head might not negotiate the mother's pelvis during labour. There had been no discussion of this at all, and I had had experience of a similar, but not identical, problem.

The head had been safely delivered, and my fingers went down the foetal neck to check that it was free of umbilical cord. All was well. Now the shoulders had to be delivered. I found that they would not move. At that moment, the Obstetric Registrar, Dr T., entered the room, and quickly summed up the situation.

'Miss Percy, I am going to put my arms around your waist and pull. You control the shoulders. We will work together.'

There was an almighty heave and the body of the baby emerged. I noted that the infant's shoulders were vast, not unlike those of a rugby player.

Mrs P. was admitted to the Antenatal Ward because her abdomen was much more swollen than it should have been for that stage of her pregnancy. On carefully palpating the abdomen, the consensus was that this was not twins, but an increased volume of liquid in the uterus. The only diagnostic modality available was X-Ray, and while we left for afternoon lectures, Mrs P. departed by ambulance for the X-Ray department at the Central City Hospital.

Next morning, the ward round was conducted by the Professor. We visited Mrs P. and pleasantries were exchanged without further discussion about her condition. When the door to her room was closed, the Professor silently indicated that we were all to move to the bottom of the unit where there was a teaching area.

'You are all aware that, yesterday, Mrs P. had an X-Ray of her abdomen. It showed that the foetus has no skull and will have no brain above the brain stem. This is the most severe neural tube defect and is called anencephaly. This foetus will not survive delivery. I am going to speak to her and her husband after the ward round. Are there any questions?'

'Now that we know that this foetus is severely abnormal and will not survive, when will steps be taken to bring this pregnancy to a conclusion?'

The Professor slipped his gold half-moon spectacles to the end of his nose and glared at me.

'Miss Percy, what you have just suggested is illegal. This conversation is finished.'

The pregnancy was to go to term, with Mrs P. carrying a foetus that would not survive. I found this decision illogical, and completely lacking in compassion.

Student accommodation at the Central Woman's Hospital was purpose built and known to us as Chorionic Villa after a tissue in the placenta. During a period of residence in the summer, a problem patient was admitted. It had been difficult to monitor the pregnancy because of her size. The scales in the Antenatal Clinic went up to twenty stone and broke. The vegetable scales in the hospital kitchen were similarly unhelpful, as they only went up to twenty-five stone. She was in excess of this. The hospital wards were in layers, with gynaecology wards sandwiched above and below obstetric wards. Outpatients were on the ground floor. When this patient walked down the corridor, we were all aware of it.

As there was grave concern for the wellbeing of the foetus, it was decided that immediate delivery by caesarean section was necessary, on a Sunday afternoon. Two Senior Registrars would perform the operation. Gowned and masked, I was asked to position myself immediately behind the surgeon, who gave the following instruction:

'Miss Percy, I want you to part my operating gown at the back and get a firm grip on the hem of my operating shirt. There is no way I am disappearing into this abdomen.'

The Professor may have had a greater interest in Gynaecology than in Obstetrics. A serious wound infection was treated successfully with honey, 'such a strong sugar solution, no bug will survive', and an abnormal channel between the urinary bladder and vagina closed with a silver stitch.

Chapter Eleven

The Children's Hospital was in the centre of the university buildings and opposite an attractive park which contained a large domed Victorian glasshouse. The student residence rejoiced in the soubriquet Fillpot Chambers. Unique among the residences, it had a snooker table. Small persons who were not ill enough to be confined to bed or cot could be a handful – one such individual was Arthur. He had congenital heart disease, and associated facial abnormalities. Full of mischief, he needed constant attention, and on one occasion I discovered him about to insert the points of metal scissors into a live electrical socket.

One of the cots held a baby boy who was nursed in a seat, never flat. He was distinguished from all the other babies by a small ball of cotton wool on each side of his head, at the top. A collection of blood had formed under the fibrous membrane covering the brain, which was drained daily with a needle, hence the cotton wool. He resembled a startled rabbit. I became involved in his care while doing the necessary paediatric nursing course that was part of our instruction. I continued to visit the Children's Hospital on Wednesday afternoons to feed him and play with him after my paediatric attachment ended. During one of these visits I overheard the following exchange between the paediatric registrar and Sister:

'Does she know the background, and that this is almost certainly a BB?'

'We are unsure whether she knows or not, but it is important that this baby has some affection in his life.'

A BB was a battered baby. Did he survive? He would be middle-aged by now.

Every day the consultant paediatricians had a ward round at 5pm, where they saw each other's cases. This was a most useful teaching opportunity for junior doctors and medical students. Sometimes there were international visitors on the Grand Round. The patient was a pale, listless girl of about eighteen months of age. Various diagnoses were suggested and plans for investigation considered. Consultant Dr J.B, himself pale in complexion, remained silent. The entourage reached the Seminar Room and discussion of the patients seen in the ward round began. After ten minutes, in which Dr J.B had sat with an abstracted expression on his face, he suddenly spoke:

'I know what is wrong with that girl. She has lead poisoning.'

It was pointed out that lead had been excluded from paint, the usual source, for a long time, but he persisted.

'She has lead poisoning.'

And so, it proved. The little girl was not her parent's first born, and the father had decided that he would repaint the cot. As the job would not take a lot of paint, he had used the remains of a tin that he had found in the garden shed. All was well at first, until the child began to gnaw at the bars of the cot.

The Children's Hospital had a significant interest in spina bifida as there was a raised incidence of the condition in the area. Clinical material for research was stored in the grounds of the hospital annexe in what was a very wealthy area to the West of the city. The Edwardian mansion had been built with commodious stables and carriage houses. We visited for inpatient ward rounds. At the end of one of these rounds, we were taken to a carriage house where a number of tall black dustbins were stored. There was an overpowering smell of formaldehyde when the top of one was removed, and within the liquid were eight rounded shapes. These were the skull convexity of children who had died from spina bifida. The whole central nervous system had been removed en bloc for research when a suitable research fellow could be recruited and funded.

As part of our paediatric surgical experience, we were to present ourselves at one of the operating theatres to see Mr S. perform a surgical procedure of his own devising to help child patients with spina bifida. Surgeons came from all over the world to see this performed. Mr S. had given a tutorial on his procedure in which he explained that if the hip could be made stable, a child could walk with callipers, instead of being confined to a wheelchair. To stabilise the hip, one of the big muscles which normally acted to bend it (psoas major) would be detached from the upper thigh bone together with the bony prominence into which it was inserted. The muscle and the prominence would then be moved to the back of the hip and reattached with two metal staples. Now, when the muscle contracted, the hip would straighten instead of flex; in this straightened position, weight bearing could occur.

We students, masked and gowned, stood behind Mr S. as he operated. He was an extremely skilled surgeon, and as he worked, he fired unrelenting questions at the junior staff. He reserved questions on the anatomy of the hip joint, the surrounding muscles and their blood and nerve supply for we students – and we had not had recourse to this knowledge for two years. When my turn came, the question was:

'Give me the branches of the lateral circumflex femoral artery.'

I began, 'Ascending, descending, and . . .'

'TOO SLOW. Ascending, descending and transverse, and don't you EVER forget it.'

I never did.

The Professor of Paediatrics ensured that we all gained a thorough knowledge of how the normal child develops from babyhood, through schooling, to adolescence. His knowledge was renowned, but, after much observation and discussion, we students concluded that we were not certain he actually liked children at all.

The girl's mother was apologetic.

'I don't like to trouble the hospital, but she insists that something is wrong. When we were on holiday I took her to the hospital where we were. Sister had a look and said there was nothing to find.'

Her daughter was ten years old, and insistent that she had something in her eye. She was quite confident to get into the large black examination chair in the eye cubicle, and tilt back her head while the inspection light was adjusted to focus on the problem area. Once the eye was properly illuminated, the culprit was obvious. At the junction between the blue iris and white sclera of the eye, at five o'clock position, there was a small pronounced bulge. The mother was called over to see what good light had revealed. Local anaesthetic drops were then instilled into the eye and given time to take effect. It was not difficult to remove the offending piece of grit with the appropriate instrument, but quite a deep ulcer, surrounded by a fibrous reaction, was left behind. A pad was placed upon her eye until the local anaesthetic wore off, and an appointment was made for the next consultant eye clinic. A cursory look is no good for a suspected foreign body.

As students, our exposure to problems of the ear, nose and throat was limited, but two female patients made a lasting impression on me. The first was referred to Mr Y., the ENT surgeon, by her general practitioner because of a lump in the right tonsil, for which diagnosis and treatment were requested. One by one we peered into the mouth of this lady and proffered various opinions. Very few in our group of eight had bothered to read the small recommended textbook on ENT, but I had a copy. The slim volume was well devised and easy to read. When my turn came, I ventured a diagnosis, stating that the beige coloured mass was a tonsillar concretion arising from debris in one of the crypts of the tonsil. Mr Y. picked up a metal probe to dislodge this stinking yellowish lump out of the crypt, and instructed the patient to use the handle of a toothbrush to express any that would form in the future. No further treatment was necessary.

The second patient was a smiling middle-aged lady with beautifully arranged hair and a string of pearls around her neck. Mr Y. had operated on her for cancer of the middle ear and she was delighted with the result. She felt very well and was enjoying life.

Six weeks later, she returned to the clinic in agony. The cancer had returned and she was devastated. She succumbed quite quickly.

Lectures from the Home Office Pathologist were a delight, delivered with aplomb and always of interest. Throughout my undergraduate career, I always sat in the third row of the central section in a stepped lecture theatre, as to my mind, that position gave the best view of the blackboard or screen if slides were to be projected. As the course in Forensic Medicine proceeded, we worked our way through murder with various agents, suicide, infanticide and other related issues of sudden death. An image particularly remembered was of the leather boots worn by a cricketer who had been struck by a bolt of lightning. Delicate branching burns, like the outlines of a feather, laced the surface of each boot, left behind by the bolt as it travelled down to earth through the player's body.

One lecture concluded with the announcement:

'Ladies and Gentlemen, next week we will be moving on to Sexual Deviancy.'

Before the appointed time the following week, a queue had formed on the stairs to the lecture theatre. Individuals not normally known for their diligence and enthusiasm for learning had made a rare appearance. My usual seat was unlikely to be available, and so it proved. Those who were normally absent had made a beeline for the front seats. As usual, an instructive lecture was given and we entered information into our notebooks. The lights were lowered for images to be projected onto the screen, and I grew bemused. One slide showed four men, but I could not work out quite what was going on before the next image appeared.

At one of our five yearly reunions, after graduation, the Home Office Pathologist was a guest lecturer. He showed us that same image. I was still unsure of the linkage – and perhaps it was better that way!

Chapter Twelve

The last year of our course, which would lead to Part Three finals and graduation, consisted of Medicine, Surgery and Psychiatry, building on the clinical experience of year IV. One of my medical attachments was with Dr Stone at the Northern Hospital. He was at pains to get the eight students on attachment to his firm to perfect their clinical technique. Having watched me percuss the chest of a patient, as I listened for the dull sound that would indicate that the lung beneath the fingers was not filled with air, he asked where I had practised my technique. On learning that I had trained on a wooden table in my flat, I was asked to remember that I was assessing a human being and *not* a piece of furniture.

On one of his ward rounds, he pointed out a male patient who was seated on a wheelchair in the centre of the ward. This man's bed had been stripped to the frame for thorough cleansing by the Nurses, as he had been discharged and was now waiting for transport to take him home. Dr Stone explained that he had been treated very successfully for Pernicious Anaemia with injections of Vitamin B12 and had recovered well. My scepticism was detected.

'Out with it, Miss Percy, say what you think.'

'I do not think there has been any success, if he is still in a wheelchair.'

Dr Stone looked across to the central table in the ward.

'Mr M., Miss Percy is not impressed by your treatment, as you still require assistance to move; just show her!'

With that, Mr M. stood up and walked the length of the ward with comparative ease.

As students in our Final Year, we were becoming rather fond of most of the consultant physicians on our attachments, with one notable exception: the Professor of Medicine. Of average height, with a balding head and gold-rimmed glasses, he had an intense gaze that one hoped fervently never to encounter. He was known as The Smiling Tiger, and we were very wary of him.

It was during final year that disposable sterile plastic equipment became available. Taking blood was much easier with the butterfly needle, which had a plastic flange at each side of the needle base, to be gripped while puncturing a vein. Leading from this area was a short, narrow length of clear plastic tubing, and then an orifice which fitted the nozzle of the, by then, plastic syringe. The flanges were held in place with adhesive tape. Each system was used once only, and the short needle always had a sharp tip. The days of resharpening steel needles were over.

Liquids for infusion were now in transparent sterile plastic bags, not glass bottles. Each bag had a thickened rounded plastic area at the base, with a central foramen for suspension from the drip stand. The metal cradle was now obsolete. A new sterile system for long term infusion of fluids also appeared. This had a central sharp sterile needle surrounded by a blunt-tipped plastic sheath. Once the device was in a vein, it could be advanced, and then the steel central needle was drawn, leaving the blunt-tipped cannula in place. Infusions could occur for days through this system.

Practicing with both of these devices was easy; we all had veins!

The students' residence at the central city hospital – the aforementioned Bedside Manor – was at the south-east corner of the hospital site, opposite The Prince of Wales pub. Built on three floors, with lockers at ground floor level, the first floor had a kitchen with a hatch into the dining room. This opened into a sitting room with a black and white television set. There was one bedroom on this floor. The second floor had twin-bedded rooms and a bathroom. Three maids were employed to clean, cook breakfast, serve lunch and wash up. A trolley arrived from the hospital containing the food for lunch; dinner was eaten in the students' dining room on the first floor of the hospital, off the main corridor.

The maids were middle-aged women who came in from home, M, D and P. M was petite and in her late forties. Her light brown hair was parted at the side, tightly curled around her ears and towards the nape of her neck, suggestive of her having used old-fashioned metal curlers. She had bright blue eyes, almost invariably illuminated with eyeshadow of a similar hue, and offset with vivid red lipstick. Mascara was liberally applied. She was a diligent worker with a good level of repartee. D was taller and older, with short dark hair and a slightly upturned nose. She took no nonsense from anyone, but had a mischievous sense of humour. Tallest and quietest of the three was P. She was mousy-haired with grey eyes, which were sheltered behind colourless NHS spectacle frames. She formed the filling in the sandwich, fitting neatly between her colleagues. Everyone respected the maids.

During our final year, P unexpectedly left in mysterious circumstances which were not discussed. She was replaced by a large West Indian lady who was firmly of the opinion that the most effective way to deal with greasy plates was with cold water and lashings of detergent. The results of this regimen were loudly scorned by M and D, and so the replacement for P disappeared. Hot water for washing up resumed with the second replacement.

The local Press revealed the cause of P's sudden departure. Her husband had an interest in photography, which he practised in a locked room of the marital home. Only he had a key. The age of his subjects, and the type of image he favoured, brought him to the attentions of H.M. Police Force. Rumour had it that he died in prison.

The single bedroom on the first floor of Bedside Manor was always sought after, as it was tucked away from the other rooms. In final year, two students were conducting an affair, and when the list of clinical teams were released, there was changing of places so that they could be together. When in residence, the male always commandeered the single bedroom. This irritated the rest of us, and we decided that sabotage would be a lark.

Acting together, with a lookout, we orchestrated a series of apple pie beds using a variety of ingredients, from sugar to holly leaves. It was decided that we would make the last night at Bedside Manor, before our final examinations began, a spectacular one. We wanted to make sure that the female student would be unable to leave the first-floor single bedroom, to stop her from haring upstairs to where she should have been, before the maids arrived in the morning. This would involve waiting until the two lovebirds were ensconced in the single room, then creeping downstairs and unscrewing the handle of the door. In the early morning, the door would therefore not open from the inside. The handle and screws were left on the lowermost stair for the maids to find. There was to be a total embargo on the identity of those involved.

It worked brilliantly.

That afternoon, the year assembled for lectures. With fifteen minutes to spare, the love birds arrived and the male strode up to the podium.

Incandescent, he started to rant about the sabotage of the bedroom, culminating in the removal of the door handle.

'No one has had the guts to own up to this and apologise, but I know full well who is responsible. It is you, Alec South, but you daren't admit it.'

No one spoke. The pact of silence held, and held for forty-five years.

Chapter Thirteen

In late spring, early summer of final year, I had a three-month psychiatric attachment to a clinic towards the west of the city. It was close to the Neurology and Plastic Surgery Annexe, and my morning walk followed the same route through the city parks. Walking through raised beds of wall flowers and tulips was a joy.

As with all clinical attachments, students had to be ready for work at 9am, dressed in a white coat with a name badge, valuables in one pocket and notebook and pen at the ready. We gathered in the entrance foyer of the clinic, talking quietly. At nine o' clock sharp, a male charge nurse appeared. He was about 5ft 8 inches tall, with dark hair worn in a side parting. Solidly built, he wore a white tunic top like a battle dress, with epaulettes, matching white trousers and black shoes. In his hand was a sheet of paper with the names of the patients chosen by the consultant psychiatrist to be clerked by us. One by one, each student was given the name of a patient and told where that person could be found. The foyer of the psychiatric clinic began to empty, until the charge nurse and I were alone.

'Right, Miss Percy, your patient is in this room,' his voice lowered. 'A word of warning. Do not, DO NOT, let him get between you and the door. I will be right outside.'

The door was of white painted wood, with a thick glass window in the upper fifth section of it. As I knocked and entered, Charge Nurse took up his position outside.

At the far side of the room sat a man of twenty-five to thirty years of age. I saw bright auburn wavy hair, deep blue eyes, and a fresh complexion. With an abiding interest in history, one name came immediately to mind: Lucius Domitius Ahenobarbus Nero. I was familiar with the face of the emperor from his coinage.

'Good morning Mr X,' I began, 'I am Miss Percy, a final year medical student. Are you willing to answer some questions and talk to me?'

He readily agreed and we walked towards a small table with a chair either side. I selected the chair nearest to the door, and glanced up at the window as I took my seat. The charge nurse was still outside. A routine clerking began, with the recording of the patient's name, address, date of birth and occupation. All information received was written down in a spiral-bound notebook. Mr X began relating the account of his present complaint, and the blank lines of the notebook filled up rapidly with my handwriting in blue ballpoint pen. Eventually, both speaker and transcriber were aware that the bottom line of the page was almost completed. Mr X stopped talking, and I placed my pen on the table to turn over.

As I did so, the atmosphere in the room changed. I looked up into a pair of icy blue eyes. The man was staring at me fixedly.

'You have a very *little* neck.' he observed.

I thought to myself, 'Well done Anona, you have managed to get yourself into a room with the neighbourhood strangler – or someone with the intentions of becoming so. Get this interview under control, NOW.'

I placed both hands on top of my notebook, and gently intertwined my fingers.

'I do know about my neck, but you see, I have the most incredibly strong hands.'

It was like flicking a light switch. He reverted to his previous demeanour and the interview continued to the close without incident. Charge Nurse was still outside when I left the room.

What I said to that patient was a complete lie. My grip is weak, like that of my mother, and a gadget is necessary for me to even remove the tops of jars and bottles. I decided that the most effective method of getting the interview back on track was to claim dominance, and fortunately, it worked.

We were now experienced at drawing blood and clerking patients. When in residence for surgery, we accompanied patients to the operating theatre. We were wary of the theatre sisters, but respected them greatly for the discipline they applied to their work.

This iron discipline should have continued into the night with emergency cases. The patient was a very overweight man with a pendulous belly, who had developed an obstruction of the small bowel. Once the abdomen was opened, the incision filled with abdominal contents, and it proved difficult to maintain a clear field of vision even with the assistant surgeon holding two retaining instruments in place. The cause of the obstruction was identified by the senior registrar Mr D., and a difficult closure was obtained. The patient was discharged home after seven days.

Sometime later, he was readmitted with another obstructive episode and it was decided to request an X-Ray image of his abdomen. This image revealed a swab left behind during the initial operation. A rule was quickly initiated, stipulating that no swab was to enter the open abdomen unless it was securely gripped in the jaws of an instrument. Sister was responsible for counting out all packs of swabs, and those that had been used were hung up on a frame with steel hooks in the operating theatre. The count out by Sister and the count of swabs on the frame by Theatre Nurse had to tally before the abdomen was closed. Large fabric packs, like men's handkerchiefs, all had a long tape at one corner, which lay around the incision to signify the presence of the pack within.

Mr L. was referred by his General Practitioner to Mr W., a urologist, or specialist in the kidneys, ureters and bladder. The patient had complained of loss of appetite and weight, and a swelling could be felt at the back of the abdomen on the left-hand side. An X-Ray examination to demonstrate the internal structure of the kidneys had shown that the left kidney was not functioning. Further information on this was required and Dr G, a consultant radiologist, was going to perform a specialised examination of the blood supply to that kidney. The student team descended to the hospital basement, which housed the Radiology department. Dr G. explained how he was going to get a long plastic tube through a steel needle in the major artery to the left leg, in front of the hip joint. The tube would then be passed up to the kidney region and a rapid series of X-Ray images would be taken, as a liquid containing iodine – which would show up on the images – would be injected down the left renal artery.

Those in the room had to wear heavy lead aprons to protect their organs from the radiation. Those without aprons had to stand behind a protective lead screen. When the X-Ray images were developed, small new blood vessels showed up around the site of the non-functioning left kidney, and we were told that this new vessel formation was one of the features of kidney cancer.

Both the consultant Mr W. and his Senior Registrar were in theatre for the removal of Mr L's left kidney. Sister had a wide trolley covered with instruments, and there were three stands to display the used swabs and packs on their hooks. The patient was positioned on his right side on the operating table, with his right hand above his head. The table was then raised into a peak beneath the upper part of the abdomen, so that the chest and head were slightly depressed. We students kept well back out of the way until we were spoken to.

Mr W. made a large incision and then mobilised the mass. He placed metal clamps on the left renal artery and vein, before dividing them and tying off the vessels. The mass was then placed in a large steel bowl and handed to me with the instruction: 'Take this into the Prep Room and divide it with this knife. I will come in a minute and see what it looks like inside.'

This prompted an outburst from Theatre Sister.

'Mr W., nothing leaves this theatre until I have checked that there is not a swab associated with it, and you KNOW that!'

There was an abject apology, the specimen was checked by Sister, and then removed to the Prep Room. The knife I wielded did not reveal cancer, but an organ that was totally replaced by pus. The mass was a huge abscess, the stench of which pervaded all around.

A second period of residence in surgery was at an older hospital in a less favoured area of town, right on the floor of the river valley around which the city had grown. In the past, the building was once a workhouse. The medical students' residence was on a hillside above the hospital, and known to decades of students as Charcot's Joint, named after a syphilis-related joint affliction. It had originally been a three storey Victorian villa, and may well have been desirable when it was constructed. With the passing of the years and the bombing of the Second World War, the surrounding neighbourhood had gone downhill and there was a lot of surrounding demolition. The hospital was surrounded by a stone wall and, at night, only one of the gates was open for entry. This gate was furthest away from the student residence on the hillside. When alerted to an emergency admission during the night, the route taken involved climbing over the wall adjacent to the hospital coke heap. We then had to clamber over the coke and enter the complex of the buildings from there – it saved valuable time.

By the late Sixties, the coke-fed boiler in the cellar at Charcot's was unreliable. It was supplied with fuel during the evening by the male students, as rats had taken up residence in the cellar. During a period of residence in final year, the boiler finally broke down completely and there was snow on the ground. The ward sisters did their best by providing us with extra blankets, but after two cold, sleepless nights, I decided to travel to my flat by the last bus, and then return by the first bus in the morning. That way I could get some sleep.

When the bill arrived for the period of residence, I paid for all the food, but for two night's lodging only, providing an explanation as to why I was not paying for the rest. This failure to pay was notified to the Dean of Medicine, who contacted the President of the Medical Student's Society. The President knew all about my failure to pay and the conditions at Charcot's that had precipitated it. His opinion was that any attempt to recover the debt, which was small, would reflect badly on the hospital and the Faculty of Medicine, especially if the conditions in which medical students were being accommodated were to become generally known.

It was during a period of residence at Charcot's that comparisons were made one evening with Fillpot Chambers at the Children's Hospital. One of the men pointed out, with some vehemence, that they even had a snooker table. It was decided that, to improve matters somewhat at Chorionic Villa, it would be a good idea to liberate the snooker table from Fillpot Chambers during the night. Four of the men made their way up the hill to the Children's Hospital in the early hours of the morning, and brought the snooker table out through one of the downstairs windows. Goodness knows how they were not either seen or heard. They then pushed the table into the middle of an empty road, and down the hill to Charcot's.

In the October of our final year, the surgical ward round was coming to an end. Each bed had been visited and the progress of the patient had been described following their surgery, which had taken place a few days previously. Some patients were delighted to be told that, as their guts were making noises again, a light diet could be started. Others were not so lucky and remained on an intravenous drip with a tube from nose to stomach, as the small bowel was not yet active. Dressings were removed and wounds inspected; further measures could be prescribed for the area. Instructions were given on the partial removal of stitches. When all this had been completed for the final patient, the consultant asked him if there was anything that he wished to add. While the ward round was in progress, he had been listening surreptitiously to a transistor radio through tiny headphones.

'There has been a catastrophe in South Wales,' he announced, 'A primary school has been engulfed by colliery waste and many children are dead. They are still digging for possible survivors.'

In this way, we learned of Aberfan.

The Orthopaedic Clinic was always of interest, as we saw so many different abnormalities. Over the period of attachment, we could assess what surgery could do to improve the mobility, and the life, of the patient. One patient taught me a lesson which was never forgotten.

She was in her early fifties and had sustained an open fracture of the lower leg, and infection had set in. A thick stench preceded her arrival in a wheelchair, with her leg extended in front of her on a board. The consultant spent a long time discussing possible future treatment with her. The reek from her leg was beginning to make some of us gag. She looked across the room at us, and spoke quietly.

'Please remember, I have this all the time. You can get away from it.'

Those who were fortunate enough to watch the spinal surgeon DKE operate were in awe of his skill. His manipulation of a broken or dislocated neck was masterful, but I never witnessed it. I only remember his face.

Chapter Fourteen

During our training, the Dean of Medicine gave a course on the history of the subject and introduced us to Galen, the Hunter Brothers, Louis Pasteur and the work of Lord Lister. We had no further contact with him until just before our final examinations.

His lecture on Medical Ethics was understood by us all to carry a three-line whip. The lecture theatre filled early, and some students were sitting on the stairs. Everyone rose as the Dean entered and resumed their seats at his invitation.

'Ladies and Gentlemen,' he began. 'You will soon be sitting the examinations which I am confident that you will pass if you have been diligent in your studies. A pass will enable the University to confer upon you the degree of Bachelor of Medicine, Bachelor of Surgery, MB, CH.B. However, in order to practise Medicine, your name and qualification needs to be registered with the General Medical Council. The University will obtain Provisional Registration on your behalf. After one year, consisting of two six-month periods of hospital practice in a medical and surgical discipline, you will be eligible for full registration, for which a fee is payable. An annual fee is then necessary to maintain your registration, without which you cannot practise.

'It is most important that you understand that the General Medical Council can revoke your registration for conduct unbecoming to a registered medical practitioner. Any conviction of a member of the profession in the law courts is automatically notified to the GMC. In particular, attention is paid to three issues, which are easy to remember as each one begins with the letter 'A'.

The first is addiction. Every year there are medical practitioners who lose their livelihood because of it. Two branches of the profession are more at risk than others because of easy access to drugs. They are firstly general practitioners, who of necessity must have controlled drugs available for their patients. The second group are anaesthetists. Other doctors needing access to this group of drugs will be closely monitored and observed. Addiction to tranquillisers is also easier to facilitate for GPs. Alcohol is something to be wary of. No patient will want to consult a doctor with a reputation for regular inebriation or smelling of alcohol. You have been warned. Convictions for drunk and disorderly conduct are not looked upon with favour by the GMC.

'Adultery with a patient is a very serious breach of trust, not only of the patient, but of the whole family. You have access to the home and medical history of the patient. To betray that trust is behaviour that the profession will not condone. You are warned!

'The last of the A's is advertising, a subject much frowned upon by the profession, and we *are* a profession, not a trade selling motor cars or hardware. Those of you who enter general practice may display a brass or other plate bearing your name and qualifications, but NOTHING ELSE. If you are invited to attend a community event in a medical capacity your name is not to be mentioned in speech or print, only that a doctor is in attendance. This also applies to involvement with radio and television.

'In dealings with professional colleagues you are unfailingly courteous, even if, privately, you consider the other party to be an absolute fool. Robust opinion or criticism is only voiced in private, where all hearers are members of the profession.

'For those of you who go on to be consultants in hospital practice, to be referred a colleague or a member of staff in the National Health Service as a patient is an honour, and is never, ever, delegated. You operate yourself on colleagues and other members of staff. In doing so, you will not only fulfil your professional obligations, but you will also begin to create your own legend.

'Do not dabble. If you have specialist training as a chest physician do not decide to begin to treat patients with Colitis. The patient will suffer for your ignorance.

'It goes without saying that colleagues and NHS staff are never used for teaching purposes. No patient is ever used for teaching without being asked their consent – basic manners, Ladies and Gentlemen.

'What you are told by a patient during a consultation is only divulged to those who need to know, for example, when arranging a further referral or investigation. Patients must have the assurance of complete confidentiality, and that sensitive matters will not be divulged to family – theirs or yours, or to other people.

'When finals are over, I trust that the Graduation Ceremony involves each one of you. Good afternoon, Ladies and Gentlemen.'

Chapter Fifteen

In each of the final year subjects, there was a rigorous examination in June. Each discipline set two written papers: there was a clinical examination involving selected patients, and an oral examination. Both the clinical and oral examination could involve an examiner from another university. It was quite possible to get a difference of opinion between the assessors in a clinical examination, which often led to them moving away from the patient and student – matters could get quite heated. Oral examinations produced widespread anxiety. The most feared one was a viva on surgical instruments. We had limited experience of the operating theatre, and great concerns about what might be asked.

As candidates, the time and site of the examination had to be determined. This meant arriving well before 9am to ascertain which alphabetical system was being used, starting from A or Y (No student in our year had a surname that began with Z). The Department of Surgery was using three adjacent ground floor laboratories to stage the Surgical Instruments viva, and my name was on the list for the central laboratory, in late morning. It was always wise to turn up early in case a candidate had been taken ill, or there had been a family emergency.

The whole system was controlled by the sound of one bell. This signalled the time at which a student could approach the door, knock and enter. When the bell next sounded, the examination was over and the student left the room. There would then be a pause to allow time for the examiner to enter a mark, and to add any comment onto a record sheet. The next ring heralded the imminent arrival of another candidate.

I was early enough to see the candidate two ahead of me enter the room. When he emerged, he would not look at those waiting outside, and this behaviour was repeated by the candidate immediately ahead of me. He kept his eyes on the horizon and avoided my gaze. My spirits were soothed by the thought that I was only going to answer questions from an examiner, not face a firing squad. Then the bell sounded. I walked forward, knocked on the door, and entered.

Opposite the door, the laboratory had windows from waist height to the ceiling. A bench reached the base of the glass and ran all the way around the room. It carried four microscopes at various points, and large glass jars containing pathological specimens were dotted about. The remainder of the surface, within my field of vision, was covered in surgical steel.

I could not see the examiner until I turned to close the door and found that he was standing right behind it. I was looking at the Professor of Surgery.

'Ah, Miss Percy. Listen carefully to my instructions. I want you to bend your arms at the elbow. I am going to take hold of your forearms and steer you backwards across the room. When we reach the other side, I want you to reach your hand behind you, without looking, and pick up the first instrument your fingers encounter. Identify it, and tell me when you have seen it used, and by whom. Is it that clear?'

It was very clear. I bent my elbows, he gripped my forearms, and I was steered backwards in a kind of weird foxtrot. When my bottom reached the edge of the bench on the opposite side of the room, my hand went behind me to see what I would encounter.

For some reason that I could not ascertain, the Professor appeared to become very angry. His face was flushed and his eyes flashed. I went back over the instructions he had given me in my head, and confirmed that I had indeed followed them. Whatever was wrong with the man? Maybe he was going to have a stroke, or a coronary? I decided to wait until he dropped before worrying about it.

My hand came around to the front of my body and I looked at what it had picked up.

'This is an osteotome, a bone chisel. I have seen it used by Mr S. at the Children's Hospital in an operation of his own devising, where the psoas major and the associated bony insertion to the upper femur are detached and moved to the back of the hip. The bony insertion is then attached to the femur with two metal staples. This transforms the action of the muscle from a flexor to an extensor of the hip. It enables children born with spina bifida to walk with callipers instead of spending life in a wheelchair.'

'You have seen this operation performed?'

'Oh yes Professor,' I replied, 'Surgeons come from all over the world to see Mr S. operate.'

'And you have seen them?' His voice was sharp.

'Yes, and spoken to them.'

My replies did not go down well – his anger was unabated.

'For the remainder of this examination I want you to begin your answer the moment I stop speaking. Is that clear? The moment.'

I said that I understood very well. He was still incensed.

Question and answer started afresh. As usual, the initial questions were straightforward, but as time passed, they became more searching. Eventually, I paused momentarily for thought before giving my response.

In that very brief interval, there was a severe pain in the right side of my chest. The Professor had not replaced the osteotome, which had just made forceful contact with my right ribs. Surgeons have strong forearms and hands, and this one was livid. This behaviour continued until the bell sounded and I was able to leave the room.

I was sharing a one-bedroom flat with a postgraduate student at this point, and during exam season, our paths crossed little. Her working day began at 9am, but laboratory work often kept her late. Examinations never started at nine, as time was needed to set things up. The earliest ones took place at nine-thirty. Clinical examinations could be at any point in the working day. None took place on Saturday, and on Friday evening I was getting ready for sleep. My bed was positioned on the wall nearest the door, and my flat mate was sitting on hers, which was adjacent to the window wall.

'What on earth have you done to your chest?' She demanded. 'You are black and blue.'

I explained what had happened with the Professor and the osteotome.

'Anona, you *are* going to complain to the Dean?'

'No, I intend to graduate, and it would be my word against his. I would not be believed.'

My chest was still sore when I presented myself for my oral examination in Psychiatry. One examiner had given an excellent lecture course to us, while the other was the external assessor from Manchester, and unfamiliar. I was anticipating questions on the major psychiatric conditions: schizophrenia, manic depressive psychosis, and depression, both acute endogenous and reactive. As well as being familiar with the recommended standard text books, I had read extensively around the subject. The question from the internal examiner was a surprise, nevertheless.

'Talk to me about the psychological and psychiatric manifestations of multiple sclerosis.'

This was neither the time nor the place to voice my immediate thought that the question was outside the syllabus. I had clerked a number of patients with multiple sclerosis in both Medicine and Neurology, however, and managed to speak sensibly until the bell sounded the end of the first half of the examination.

What would the external examiner produce after that? Surely something straightforward?

'Talk to me about the causes and treatment of impotence in a man of thirty-four years of age.'

I did not remember that in the syllabus either. However, information from Medicine, Surgery, Pharmacology and the women's magazines I had encountered came together, and I had not finished all I considered necessary in my answer when the bell sounded for the end of the examination. I heard it, and so did both of the assessors. The external examiner, however, was determined to continue.

'I realise that you have not completed your response to my question, however I have to mention this topic: what about Sunday afternoon?'

The bell had rung, the examination was over. Nothing I said now would make any difference to my mark, and this man was beginning to irritate. I began to rise from my chair.

'Is Sunday afternoon a request for additional information regarding my response to your question, or an invitation?'

I left the room to the sound of delighted male laughter.

The schedule for final examinations was drawing to a close. The last, a viva in Medicine, was held on a sunny June afternoon. The weather was fine, and I was wearing a cotton dress and wool cardigan under my white coat.

I only recall one examiner from this viva. Yet again, I had drawn the external examiner, and it was Professor S.S. from London, an expert on the liver. The early questions were very straightforward as usual, and required little in the way of thought. Then, a more involved topic:

'Talk to me about the causes and treatment of kidney failure.'

This was a vast subject, and one that had been thoroughly researched and rehearsed. It gave the opportunity to speak sensibly while looking elsewhere except at the examiner. On the table between us was a large sheet of white paper, with a broad column on the left of the examiner which contained two words on each line. Travelling to the right were narrow columns of figures. The column on the extreme right only held five sets of figures in the spaces from the top.

As I continued to speak about renal failure, the piece of paper began to move slowly across the table towards me. I realised that I was looking at all the examination marks to date, upside down. As the column on the extreme right, my left, held only five sets of figures in the spaces from the top, I realised that I must be the candidate on line six. My name is easy to read upside down because of the 'Y' at the end. The hunch was correct and my eyes travelled horizontally towards my left, reading my marks. I had scored a very safe pass. The paper then began to slowly retreat across the table to the examiner. The bell sounded the end of my examination before I had completed all I had to say on renal failure.

'Every good wish for your future career.'

'Thank you, Professor.'

With that, I left the room knowing that all was well, and I was going to graduate in Medicine.

The Borders Hospital

HOUSE JOBS

Following graduation, I decided that my first pre-registration post would be in Medicine. It was away from the city of my undergraduate training.

The Borders Hospital was built on a gently sloping site to the east of a market town in the south of England. Originally constructed to cope with casualties of the First World War, it nestled among an area of desirable detached houses. It was surrounded by trees, many of which were conifers. The main hospital was single storey, with wards on either side of a sloping central corridor. Each ward bore the name of a cathedral city. Near the bottom of the slope, on the left, was the operating theatre. A second theatre for fracture and dislocation reduction and resuscitation was available in the Accident and Emergency Department. The hospital shop, selling newspapers, magazines and confectionery, was to the right of the corridor, in the centre of the slope. Off a subsidiary corridor, and at right angles to the main corridor, was the Accident and Emergency Department. This was immediately adjacent to a spacious car park.

A detached two-storey brick-built block provided facilities for psychiatric patients on the ground floor and maternity patients on the first floor. There was no lift. Any maternity patient who needed an emergency caesarean section was carried downstairs on a stretcher, then across the hospital grounds on a trolley to the operating theatre off the main corridor. No psychiatric patient was to be afforded the possibility of harm through jumping out of a first-floor window. The laboratories for Biochemistry and Pathology were in a detached modern building to the left of the hospital entrance. The mortuary and the autopsy room were discreetly screened in the north-west corner of the site.

Married medical non-consultant staff lived in a modern detached block to the west of the ward complex. Single non-consultant medical staff had bedrooms in a detached bungalow to the right of the hospital entrance. A resident's lounge and small kitchen were available, and bathrooms were shared.

At the beginning of July 1967, I began a six-month duty as House Physician to Dr Napier, a spare-boned Scot with twinkling blue eyes and a dry sense of humour. Dr Johns, who was Indian, was the Medical Assistant, a non-consultant grade. He had wide clinical experience but, despite several attempts, failed to achieve the Membership of the Royal College of Physicians (MRCP). There was no medical registrar.

Lincoln was the female ward and Gloucester was the male. Each had two senior nursing staff. Both on Lincoln were female, the Junior sister a daffy blonde called Sister Watson, the Senior a more sober, dark-haired and dark-eyed lady, Sister Richards. Gloucester, however, had Sister Kussons, from Latvia, and an Irish charge nurse, Mr Musgrave.

It was a period of rapid learning: carefully supervised, but the routine was what it had been when I was a student. Now, every morning, all the blood for laboratory tests had to be obtained from the patients by me before the ward round. It was an environment in which I felt secure in my ability to care for the patients entrusted in my charge.

On call was a different matter. It was shared between Medicine, Geriatrics, and Paediatrics. Geriatrics involved the occasional demise and death certification. Paediatrics was terrifying. The consultant paediatrician, Dr S, rightly insisted on being informed of each admission. The paediatric houseman was single and lived in the Doctor's residence. Dr Annan was always willing to help with a child who was a puzzle or very sick.

My first night on call was a warm July evening with the heady scent of nicotiana in the air from the flowerbeds in the grounds. Clad in my white coat, with name badge pinned to my lapel and bleep in a pocket, I set out at 10:30pm to do the night round, starting on Winchester, the children's ward. Across the corridor was Worcester, used for infective cases and the occasional private patient. Progressing down the slope came the geriatric wards on the left and Lincoln on the right.

As I approached the latter, Night Superintendent Sister McDermott was walking up the main corridor having begun her round at Chelmsford, the closest ward to the laboratory block. She appraised me with a sceptical eye. 'Ye Gods, it's white!'

I replied, 'Good evening, Sister.'

'I do not believe this, not only white, but English!'

It was Sister McDermott who arranged for me to be equipped with a thick woollen nurse's cape for the night round as winter approached. It was much appreciated.

Patients were in hospital for much longer at that time. Medical treatment for gastric or duodenal ulceration was six weeks of bed rest with a twenty-four-hour drip of milk into the stomach through a tube passed down from the nose. Bed rest was standard for all heart attack patients too.

A London chest physician held a weekly Outpatient Clinic and was available during that visit for consultation on problem cases. From time to time, an inpatient bed was required for those patients who were to have an examination of the bronchial tubes under general anaesthetic. Consent for this procedure was taken by the consultant, Dr Scott, in the Out-patient clinic, but a standard clerking and full examination were still mandatory. Once recovered from the anaesthetic, the patient could return home, provided someone else was driving. It was a twenty-four-hour stay, no more.

The clerking had been uneventful, and the male patient disappeared on a trolley to the operating theatre for the examination. The subsequent appearance of a very pale Dr Scott on the ward was most unusual and Sister asked me to join him in a side room. What had I missed?

Looking down the instrument in the windpipe of the patient, Dr Scott had seen a bulge into one of the major bronchi. Thinking it likely to be a tumour pushing in from the surrounding tissue, he decided to take a small sample for analysis in the Pathology laboratory. Small pincers were passed down the bronchoscope to enable recovery of the sample. The field of view flooded with blood because the bulge was due to the pulmonary artery. Dr Scott would speak to the relatives himself, as it was his responsibility alone.

The stabilisation of new diabetics was a challenge, not always helped by the patient. One such patient was Mr Mayhew, who was admitted to Gloucester ward, and his wife to Peterborough, a geriatric ward. Mr Mayhew's blood glucose readings were almost impossible to control and understand. His diet was carefully managed by the dietician and the required insulin calculated daily. Yet blood glucose readings remained high. The answer to this mystery emerged when I made a rare visit to the hospital shop for more paper tissues, and discovered Mr Mayhew raiding the confectionery section!

Autumn was passing into winter and early preparations for Christmas were underway. Each ward was provided with a beautifully iced cake from the hospital kitchen. Placed in a round tin, it sat upon another square tin which was immersed to a depth of four inches in a bucket of water. There it remained until Christmas Day. Many years before, the hospital had become infested with an omnipresent insect, the pharaoh's ant. They were in the linen, in store cupboards and in the family planning goods, where their presence was said to explain the high failure rate of contraceptive devices. When clerking a patient, it was not unusual to see a pharaoh's ant scuttle across the pillow near the head of a patient. Immersion of the supporting tin that contained the Christmas cake was essential, because they could not swim.

AC was admitted as an emergency in late November with a chest infection. In her eighties, she was petite and knowledgeable. She lived in one of the desirable villages to the east of the market town. Treatment with antibiotics and physiotherapy brought the situation under control and she was ready to be discharged. The letter for her general practitioner was written, detailing the treatment given, and I went to Lincoln ward to give it to her before she left. To my surprise and embarrassment, she informed me that she had arranged for a Christmas gift to be delivered to my home. I explained that I could not accept gifts from patients, but she continued blithely on. 'I thought that would be your reaction; hence, it will go to your home. You will receive a copy of National Geographic magazine monthly for a year, from the USA. Not the United Kingdom edition!'

I voiced my surprise as to how she had achieved this. She explained that there was a longstanding relationship with the American publication. She had been a secretary in the Valley of the Kings, Egypt, when Howard Carter discovered the tomb of Tutankhamun. She had typed the original descriptions of the artefacts from the burial chambers. As Carter himself remarked, 'wonderful things.' Many years later I saw them myself in London, at the Tutankhamun Exhibition held in the British Museum.

HC was a blond, well-made young man in his early twenties. He had initially been under the care of Dr S, the Paediatrician, with kidney problems, but at the age of sixteen was transferred to Dr Napier. Recent blood and urine tests had shown that his kidneys were failing. His mother was a bustling kind of woman, with fair curly hair, who was determined to do everything in her power for her son. Dr Napier gently told her that an application had been made to the University Teaching Hospital of the region to get him accepted for renal dialysis. So far, a reply had not been received, but as soon as it arrived, he would contact the family with the result. With that, mother and son left the Outpatient Clinic. Dr Napier motioned to the nurse to delay the arrival of the next patient in the room. 'Tell me, Dr P, what was the policy on selection for dialysis in the city where you trained?' I remembered clearly a tutorial with Dr M.P, a female consultant who specialised in advanced kidney disease. Renal dialysis was available, but facilities and provision were limited, and priority was given to married men with families. Dr Napier was fairly sure that those restrictions would still apply, and that HC would not be accepted. This proved to be the case; unfortunately, his mother regarded it as a betrayal of her son, for which we, the local medical staff, were responsible.

Sister Kussons rarely discussed her homeland of Latvia. Once, she spoke about a much-respected and loved physician at the hospital in which she worked. The Nazis came, and he was Jewish. They did unspeakable things with barbed wire before they shot him. Sister rarely smiled, but when she did, it was as though the sun came out.

Onto her ward I admitted an emergency from a general practitioner. The patient was in his early thirties with a chest infection and a high temperature. It was late afternoon, and I prescribed a broad-spectrum antibiotic, Tetracycline, by mouth. Treatment began immediately, as the tablets were in stock on the ward. It was Wednesday, and my afternoon off. In the early hours of the morning I was wide awake, worrying about my choice of antibiotic. Was it really the best option? I voiced my concerns to Dr Napier before the ward round reached Gloucester. The patient did look better, and all sweating had ceased. Dr Napier picked up the temperature chart hanging at the bottom of the bed and placed it on the counterpane. It showed a rapid fall from the initial peak; my worries had been groundless.

Mr R. was admitted with a urinary tract infection which was caused by an unusual organism —Pseudomonas, not the usual E.coli. An antibiotic specifically developed for the organism had just appeared on the market, and Mr R. was receiving the medication by injection. The night round was in process and I had reached his bed.

'Dr P., those injections are doing me the power of good.'

'I'm delighted, Mr R. Each one is costing two guineas.'

He was amazed that any medication could be so expensive.

As Christmas drew nearer, extra effort was made to get as many patients as possible home to their families. Not easy, when so many conditions relied on bed rest. It was just after eleven p.m. on Christmas Eve when the general practitioner telephoned. He had an elderly lady in heart failure, who was having trouble breathing. Admission to Lincoln Ward was arranged. Night nurse placed the patient, accompanied by her daughter, in a side ward to avoid disturbing the other patients. This was just after midnight. Both ladies were disconcerted to find themselves in hospital, because the patient was not breathless at all. She had a sore throat, nothing else. On examination, the tonsils were certainly red and swollen, with a little pus in the crypts. The lymph glands in the neck were tender, but there were no other abnormal findings. All that was required was an antibiotic. The general practitioner, so eloquent on the telephone, had not seen the patient at all. Christmas Eve was not a time when he was prepared to treat a patient with tonsillitis. I began to learn about lying within the medical profession.

Chester ward was a series of separate rooms with washbasins. A heavily-built, middle aged man was admitted to one of these rooms, having had a heart attack. It was evening and the hospital was quiet as Sister McDermott entered Chester on the night round. The lamp was shining on the night nurse's desk, and it appeared from the position of the chair that she had risen rapidly to her feet. Sister knew the nurse from previous night rounds. She and her friend were very slender, attractive girls from the Far East. McDermott went on the prowl. She discovered the door of the last room standing ajar. On entering, it became obvious what had transpired. The patient had rung the emergency bell close to the bed for assistance. Nurse had run to answer it, and was bending towards the patient when he died and fell on top of her. He was heavy, and she was slight. She could not extricate herself, nor could she summon anyone to her aid. She was trapped beneath a corpse until someone entered the ward and realised that she was missing. Sister McDermott telephoned the Nurses Home and asked someone to relieve Night Nurse. The latter was dispatched to her room after a cup of tea with plenty of sugar in it, and almost certainly a tot of something alcoholic.

The Geriatric wards were a refuge for many incapacitated and frail elderly people who could not live alone. Their long stay made them familiar, and loved figures to many of the nursing staff. I was summoned to Peterborough, because Arthur had collapsed. In spite of my speedy arrival, the patient had expired. Sister was distressed. 'What are we going to do, Dr Percy? It's Arthur!' Arthur was eighty-nine years old, with chronic chest problems and a long history of little strokes. Cardiopulmonary resuscitation was most definitely not appropriate.

'I realise that the patient is special to you and the other patients on the ward, but in view of his age and underlying medical problems, resuscitation is not an option, I'm afraid. The right thing to do is telephone for a porter, when the body has been prepared, and arrange removal to the mortuary. Someone should make you a strong cup of tea and give you time to come to terms with things.'

Being on call for Paediatrics was always frightening and the passage of time did not alter this. It was a summer Sunday afternoon and a two-year-old boy was admitted with gastroenteritis. The child was very dehydrated, and when I telephoned Dr S, I said that I would cut down at the ankle to a vein and then transfuse fluid for rehydration at that point. The child was so dry that getting a drip set up any other way would have wasted time. Blood would go to the laboratory for the usual tests. All went well, but shortly after the infusion of fluid began, the child deteriorated markedly, his eyes rolling back in his head. 'Nurse, telephone Dr S and ask him to get here quickly.'

Dr S lived in a delightful half-timbered Mediaeval house in a neighbouring village. I never discovered how fast he drove to arrive as promptly as he did, but he was soon at the bedside of the child, who by now, had rallied in response to the saline drip. Later, Mr H, the Chief Laboratory Technician, ran onto the ward. 'This child has a bicarbonate level that we have never before recorded in this hospital.' Rehydration worked like magic and the little patient went home some days later. Six months as House Physician passed swiftly, and in July I began a new post at the same hospital, but in Surgery.

Mr H was approaching retirement. Balding and portly, he had a florid complexion and quizzical brown eyes. His pride and joy was his Citroen car. General practitioners in the town, having referred surgical problems to him for many years and knowing that he was winding down, were beginning to refer their cases to a new consultant surgeon, a brash Australian called Mr M. Theatre Sister had a quiet word with me about Mr M, because it was likely that at some time I would be needed to assist him. 'I need to warn you, Dr P, that Mr M throws things.' 'Really,' I replied, 'well any surgical instruments thrown at me will be promptly returned.' Word must have reached him, because he never tried it.

After each Surgical Outpatient Clinic, the waiting list came out and the patients seen in the clinic were added to the list categories. Category I were those that needed speedy attention – not urgent, but prompt. Category II patients could wait three to four weeks. Category III cases could be dealt with at any time. Each operating list was assembled around a Category I case with others selected according to the complexity of the main case.

Mrs W was a very overweight lady who had developed a pendulous flabby abdominal wall, with repeated skin infections in the folds. It was decided to remove this tissue through a wide incision above and below, to give her a flat abdominal wall which would be easy to keep infection-free. The surgery was not difficult, but as it proceeded I became aware of a wet, sticky sensation across my own abdomen. The incision was closed, and Mr H and I left the operating theatre. My surgical gown was heavily bloodstained, and when thrown into the soiled linen bin, my theatre dress beneath was in a similar state. Mr H was apologetic. 'I should have warned you to put a mackintosh apron on under the gown.' Once back in my room, all underwear had to be thrown out.

Simple surgical cases were devolved to me when I had seen the technique demonstrated and performed the same under consultant supervision. The removal of swellings on or under the skin was certainly in my domain. One such was a cyst on the back of the neck of an airline pilot. It had got to the stage of catching on the collar of his uniform tunic and I was instructed to remove it: 'Make sure you get it out intact.' Minor surgery such as this was performed in the Outpatient clinic and Sister D was to assist me.

The patient was seated with his back to me, airline tunic open and covered in surgical drapes. Having tested that the local anaesthetic that I had injected was working, I began. Soon, the cyst was deposited in a glass jar to go to the Pathology Department. The patient was informed that I was almost finished and just needed to put in some stitches. At this, he slumped in the chair in a faint. When he recovered, the necessary stitching was performed. I reported back to Mr H. 'Never operate on an upright patient, Dr P, even if it will give you the best access to the area. Always have them flat, then they cannot possibly fall.' A lesson was learned.

During the autumn, Mr H informed me that Sister D, from Surgical Outpatients, was to be admitted for drainage of a breast abscess. Examination of the area showed reddened skin but no tenderness. Her temperature was normal, as was the rest of the clinical examination.

In theatre, all was prepared for the abscess pus to go to Bacteriology, to identify the organism and the most appropriate antibiotic for it. Mr H had scalpel in hand and we were all prepared for the stench that would arise when the pus was liberated. In went the knife and nothing happened. The incision was widened, and Mr H inserted an exploratory finger to break down any fibrous tissue that might be confining the pus. His eyes registered shock. 'Oh my goodness, this is not an abscess, it's cancer.' There was a flurry of activity as we proceeded immediately to an unexpected mastectomy.

W.S Gilbert wrote: 'Things aren't always as they seem.' That is certainly true in Medicine. Examination of the tissue from this tumour under the microscope showed it to be quite a rare form of malignancy.

When in Residence on call, as there was only one operating theatre, I was available to assist other specialities who needed to use it, and was frequently requested to assist at Caesarean sections. A working relationship developed with the Obstetric/Gynaecology registrar.

Every member of the medical staff was aware of Dr W, a general practitioner in the town. He had been on the medical staff of the hospital in his younger days with a reputation for sound diagnosis. He was now in his eighties, and we had all listened to patient accounts of his methods. On his desk was a large glass jar from one of the local sweet shops, which had the adhesive label identifying the confectionery within removed. Into this jar went all samples distributed by representatives of the pharmaceutical companies – antibiotics, antidepressants, tranquillisers, and tablets for raised blood pressure. At the end of a consultation, whatever the problem, patients were dispensed a handful of goodies from this jar in a small paper bag.

A referral from Dr W was treated with extreme caution, and not admitted to any ward until assessed in A&E by the resident staff. It was Sunday afternoon, and the gynaecology registrar had just taken a call from Dr W. The patient was said to have a gangrenous prolapse of the womb. The registrar raised her eyebrows and said: 'Unusual. Come with me, Dr P, and let us see what exactly is wrong with this lady. She is coming to A&E, and I have asked the staff to get her onto the operating table so that I can examine her in a good light and see what on earth is going on.' We made our way from the Doctor's Residence across the car park to A&E, and thence into the theatre. The registrar spoke quietly to the patient and listened to her whispered replies. I could not hear what was being said. Positioning a large theatre light was a skill that I had not perfected and good lighting is essential for a gynaecological examination. I was still struggling when the registrar said: 'Dr P, get me a delivery pack quickly.' The so-called gangrenous prolapse was a foetal head with black hair and it had been in the process of arrival for some time.

Locum Consultants

At intervals, cover was required for consultants who were on holiday or sick where the speciality had only one senior practitioner. At the Borders Hospital, Pathology and Obstetrics and Gynaecology were the disciplines concerned.

There was great respect for the hospital pathologist Dr L. He was tall and quiet with white hair, and a concern for both the living and the dead. When he departed on his annual holiday, his duties were carried out by a stout middle-aged female with a rather pasty complexion. She marched between the Pathology department and the mortuary/post mortem room with a cigarette clamped between her jaws. I had not encountered a chainsmoking consultant before.

As was my practice, I attended the autopsy of a patient who had died on the ward, and then realised how fortunate we were to have Dr L. The locum pathologist smoked throughout the post mortem examination, getting the technician to light a fresh cigarette and put it in her mouth as another came to an end. The butt was deposited in any convenient body cavity that was open. Unfortunately for her, one of the deceased whose autopsy she had performed was subsequently exhumed and her butts discovered. The facts were rare enough to make the national press.

Dr Abrahams was the Consultant Obstetrician/Gynaecologist, loved and respected in hospital and town. His house was immediately outside the hospital perimeter amongst cypress trees, and he could enter the hospital grounds via a gate at the bottom of his garden. The Psychiatry/ Maternity block was the first building beyond this gate. He could sleep in his own bed and yet be available quickly if required. On occasion, he had arrived in his pyjamas. His annual holiday was of concern to many. The temporary replacement was a small man in his fifties with thin, grey greasy hair, ending in curls at ear-level. It was his practice to insist on living in the Junior Doctors' Residence. The Obstetric/Gynaecology registrar was far from pleased.

'Not him again. I remember the last time he was here. Dr Abrahams had seen a patient with heavy bleeding due to a large fibroid. She had listened carefully to what he advised and was quite willing to undergo a hysterectomy. She was in her mid-thirties, but her family was complete, and she signed the consent form for a hysterectomy in the clinic. It would however, take place when Dr Abrahams was on holiday. This locum performed the surgery and I assisted. Everything was fine until he began to remove her ovaries. I pointed out that there was no consent for this and that she would be precipitated into an early menopause. It was to no avail; he was adamant, and archly informed me that he was saving the patient from ovarian cancer. The risk of that was very small, whereas a premature menopause was inevitable. Now I have him and his practice to cope with again!'

There were other practices that we learned about. He would not eat dinner with the rest of the Mess. The kitchen adjoined the dining room and all washing up was done there. Meals arrived on a heated trolley from the hospital kitchen, but breakfast was cooked on site and was invariably fried eggs, with or without bacon. Stocks of both were in the kitchen cupboard; milk was kept in a small refrigerator. Returning to the Doctors' Mess after the night round, I saw what this individual was up to. The box of eggs and greaseproof paper-wrapped bacon was out of the store cupboard and he was cooking himself a fry-up. Not having a love of fatty foods in the morning, I was in the habit of taking with me a box of six fresh eggs when I was on call for a week. One would be boiled each morning and the box was clearly marked with my name. It was my box of eggs that he was raiding. Something had to be done!

Television was the preferred entertainment for most of the Mess at the weekend, and in the evenings. At 9:30pm, two of us took note of the preferences – tea or coffee – and would go to the kitchen to make the evening drinks. The Locum Gynaecologist wanted tea, which made the reprisal so much easier. Everyone else wanted coffee. Into the bottom of his cup went a stash of crushed laxative tablets.

Senior House Officer

I had been interested in the care and treatment of the injured since Medical School and was pleased to be selected as Senior House Officer in Accident and Emergency at the Borders Hospital. There was cross responsibility for Orthopaedics.

The hospital had no laboratory or x-ray services at night or at the weekend. The necessary staff had to be called in from home, and it had better be something important enough to do so. Wrist fractures were immobilised in a half diameter plaster cast and sent home with analgesics to return on the following day at 9am, starved. Those with probable lower limb fractures were admitted to the ward and stabilised with a system of pulleys, weights and cords known as traction. A list built up of those needing an x-ray and an anaesthetist.

In Sister's office was the red telephone which was a direct line from Ambulance Control, used to alert the department to a significant event. It rang on a hot Friday afternoon in early summer. At a notorious bend north of the market town, a sports car containing two young men had left the road and hit a tree. Would a doctor meet the ambulance in the car park?

I collected an ophthalmoscope to examine the back of the eye and made my way out into the sunshine. The wail of the ambulance siren could be heard in the far distance and the sound increased rapidly as it approached. Once stationary, one of the crew jumped out of the cab and opened the rear doors. The siren sound was now replaced by the shrieking of one of the occupants. 'Get him to the Operating Theatre now, I will be there in a minute.' The remaining young man had dark hair, smoothed straight back from his forehead, and held in place with something like Brylcream. He was motionless and ashen, with widely dilated pupils that did not react to light from my ophthalmoscope. Examination of the back of the eye confirmed death and the ambulance began its journey to the mortuary.

The other passenger, now in theatre, had light brown curly hair and very obvious multiple injuries. He was semi-conscious, shrieking continually, with both legs at appalling angles to one another and to his body. No x-ray was required to demonstrate the fractures above and below the knee. One arm was fractured below the shoulder and his pelvis was unstable on examination. I had grave doubts about his intracranial and abdominal contents.

To my surprise, the on-call anaesthetist, Dr R, arrived unsummoned. I gave him an account of the injuries that I had detected. 'Dr Percy, you must realise that the injuries are mortal.' 'I do accept that, but his parents are on their way, according to one of the nurses, and no parent should see their child with legs like that. I would like to straighten them without causing him further pain and for the nurses to be able to clean up his face and hands.' Dr R was firm but kind. 'On that basis, and on that basis alone, I will anaesthetise him, but mind, there are to be NO HEROICS.'

He went to the corner of the room and wheeled the anaesthetic machine over to the operating table. The gases were selected and then the mask gently applied to the young man's face. Before each shriek, he gulped down quantities of anaesthetic. Gradually, the volume of this sound diminished, and then all was silent. Dr R gave a nod and the nurses began to clean him up. I gently returned each section of leg to a normal position, reducing the fractures and maintaining the reduced position in a metal splint with cords attached by an adhesive tape to the skin.

There was movement from Dr R. He was pointing to the inflatable rubber bag on the anaesthetic machine which monitored the respiratory effort. It had been fully inflated with each breath, but now the respiratory effort was beginning to fail. The nurses and I had just completed our work and we stood, either side of the operating table, as his breathing slowly ceased. A nurse entered to say that his parents had arrived. Dr R wheeled the anaesthetic machine back into the corner and departed. The nurses went back to their duties and I spoke to the parents. They were shown into the operating theatre and told to spend as long as they wished with their son. Some time later, they asked to see me to express their thanks. 'It was a comfort to us to know that he was not alone at the end. The staff were there with him and we can see that he has been cared for. We are very grateful.'

Both young men were university students travelling in a sports car, going for a weekend away. Unfortunately, in a collision at high speed between a car and a tree, the occupants of the vehicle always come off worst. I can see their faces still, after almost fifty years. They were two gorgeous guys.

All head injuries that had experienced a period of unconsciousness were admitted to a ward for observation, if x-rays of the skull had revealed no fracture. Those with a fracture were referred to the Regional Neurosurgical Unit.

The House Surgeon at the time was a pretty blue-eyed and brown-haired young woman named Margaret Robertson. She was married to the Paediatric Senior House Officer.

The patient was a woman in her forties, and while examining her, both my eye and nose informed me that she was none too clean. The skull x-rays showed no fracture and Margaret agreed to admit her to a surgical bed for observation. Neither of us had concerns about the patient. Roughly a month later, virtually the whole of the Doctor's Mess was watching the Men's Final at Wimbledon on television. As the match ended, a colleague sitting opposite Margaret and me suddenly spoke up. 'I have been watching you two for some time. Do you realise that both of you are scratching your fingers?' We looked at each other and then at our hands. On both sets of hands, we detected the tell-tale burrows of scabies, probably caught from the head injury patient.

Pharmacy was closed at the weekend, but the Chief Pharmacist was a most helpful member of staff and switchboard managed to contact him at home. He was horrified. 'You both have scabies? I will come in and provide enough benzyl benzoate for you both, to cover yourselves in after a bath, on three separate days. You need fresh bed linen too. Underclothes should be soaked in the solution and then thoroughly washed.' The treatment worked, and we both stopped scratching.

I wanted more experience in trauma. Fracture and dislocation manipulation was something I found satisfying, but more examples of multiple injuries and the management of the same were required. A more central hospital would provide this. The rear pages of the British Medical Journal and the Lancet were scanned for suitable openings, one eventually arose.

The Armistice
Hospital

The Armistice Hospital was built on a site that became, over the
years, close to the ring road of a major town and a motorway.
It therefore offered the opportunity to gain more experience in
treating major trauma cases. I was keen to avail myself of all it had to
offer when I was appointed as one of the four Senior House Officers in
the Accident and Emergency Department. Of the four, one would work
a week of nights, the remaining three a changing pattern of day shifts.
The working week began on Friday, with one of us going on to night duty
and working from 5pm to 9am. At the end of that week, there would be
a weekend off. One of the three people working days would also work
on Saturday and Sunday. During the week, a more experienced female
doctor was our supervisor. The administrative control of the Department
was with the younger of the two Orthopaedic Surgeons, Mr B. This was
a much bigger medical establishment than I had previously encountered.

The Department was built on the right side of the original hospital
construction and had two entrances. That nearest the public footpath led
to a Reception Desk on the left, where patients would give particulars
and register. Female clerks then directed them into the waiting room.

Between the reception desk and waiting room was a short corridor, which led to an area with four desks at which patients could be seen by the medical staff. Beyond this area was a small examination room for eye and ear, nose and throat problems. The entrance furthest from the road was for ambulance cases and led directly to a wide corridor with six curtained areas on the right for examining and treating patients. Sister's office was on the left, opposite the first of the curtained areas.

At the far end of this corridor was the Medical Staff Office, which could be entered by a sliding door and had light boxes for x-ray images on the wall. The department had an operating theatre for fracture manipulation and minor surgery, and a busy plaster room for applying casts of Plaster of Paris. A technician was specifically employed for this and was kept busy, as there were fracture clinics to service as well as a busy Accident Department. At weekends and during the night, the medical staff applied casts themselves, which were often ridiculed by the technician and criticised by the Orthopaedic surgeons. It was most important that any cast involving the ankle kept this joint at a right angle; drooping toes were not allowed!

The X-ray Department of the hospital was close to A&E but closed at 5pm. A radiographer could be called in after hours for anything serious and, at the weekend, an agency radiographer was employed. Mrs Cox was kept very busy and no doubt the agency was well-paid by the hospital.

My first patient was a man of thirty-five years of age who worked as a butcher. I called his name in the waiting room and he followed me down to the clerking area.

'Good morning, I am Dr Percy. Please have a seat.' 'No thank you, Doctor, I prefer to stand. Sitting is very uncomfortable, and I do not feel well.'

One of the nurses escorted Mr F to one of the curtained areas to be examined, where the cause of the problem was abundantly clear. There was a large abscess on one side of his posterior.

'Mr F, when did you last eat or drink?'

'I had a cup of tea and some cereal at eight o' clock.' 'In that case, I can do nothing for you now. You have an abscess which needs draining under general anaesthetic when your stomach has emptied. I will contact the on-call anaesthetist and see when we can fit you in to have this done.' Dr H the anaesthetist arrived at 2pm, and the patient was anaesthetised on the operating table. There was no difficulty in liberating copious amounts of pus. The resultant cavity was flushed out, and then packed with ribbon gauze, leaving a protruding wick.

Once conscious, I explained to the patient that daily dressings would be required until the cavity closed up. An antibiotic was prescribed, and a sick note provided as he could not work with foodstuffs while he was infected. I saw him from time to time over the following days, and at one point he told me with delight that he could sit down again without pain.

While I was on night duty, a note was left for me stating that Mr F was enquiring about when I would next be working days. He appeared one afternoon with a large flat parcel in his hand. Over my night duty week, the abscess had healed, and he was back at work. This was not a medical visit, but a social one, and I therefore saw him away from the other patients. The parcel was presented to me with the words: 'It is a thank you Dr Percy, and I will be offended if it is not accepted.' Removing the brown paper and then opening the greaseproof paper underneath revealed eight of the largest rump steaks I had ever seen. Both medical and nursing staff profited from his generosity.

One never knew what to expect in that unit. It was a fairly busy late morning when a tall man with wavy grey hair to his shirt collar appeared in the clerking area with a baby in his arms. Two of the fingers of one of his hands were down the throat of the infant. 'I am Dr Taylor, and this child has something stuck.' Dr Taylor was a well-respected local GP whom I knew only from his referral letters. He was ushered into the small examination room for eye, throat, ears etc. and Sister D followed me in. I grabbed the Paediatric instrument for examining the throat and inserted it beneath the fingers of Dr T, which he then removed, and disappeared back to his surgery.

By the examination light, I could see a large rounded mass at the back of the mouth of this infant. I asked Sister D for a pair of dressing forceps, a gripping tool. She looked at me as if I had gone insane. 'I need them quickly Sister, there is something in here which is almost blocking the airway.' With the instrument in my hand, I got a grip on the front end of the mass and pulled. Out came a wodge of what looked like bright red paper tissue. Sister's eyebrows shot up. In went the forceps again because I had not retrieved all that was there, and once the remainder was grasped, the infant's colour began to improve from chalky grey to pale pink. The remainder of the obstruction was deposited in a steel dish. The baby went to the care of the Paediatric ward and I calmed down. The story which filtered back to me was that this very young child had eaten tissues from a box. I still wonder about that.

Weekend night shifts were usually hectic. Friday night in particular produced a variety of alcohol-induced mishaps. It was nearly midnight when the ambulance rattled up and entered with an almost comatose, heavily made-up young woman on a stretcher. Accompanying her was another female in her twenties, the worse for drink but still able to talk. She was able to identify the patient and pointed out with glee that she was getting married in the morning. The informant was one of the bridesmaids. No address could be elicited from the patient. By the time the stomach contents of the bride-to-be had been emptied into a bucket, the bridesmaid had disappeared. Night Sister and I had a name, and nothing else. The patient was a little more coherent but could not manage an understandable address. There was only one solution. There were approximately a dozen entries of that name in the only telephone directory available at the time. I had to hope that the family was not ex-directory. In the early hours of the morning, I had to make my way down the list of names, rousing people from their slumber to ask if they had a daughter getting married that day.

I struck gold on name ten. I explained who and where I was, and what had transpired. Thirty minutes later, the door of the Accident Unit was flung open, and a very angry middle-aged woman strode in and was promptly ushered behind the curtain to the bride-to-be. She was indignation personified, and after her opening salvos of criticism asked: 'What is Gordon going to say about this?' The local newspaper published photographs of the weekend brides in the Monday edition. I made a point of leaving the hospital at lunchtime to purchase a copy. The groom, Gordon, was resplendent in morning dress. His bride had her eyes half-closed but at least she was vertical.

Night Superintendent was auburn-haired, with a controlled roll of curls at her neck beneath her lace cap. When on duty, she patrolled the wards, but also the immediate environs of the hospital, dealing with the occasional drunk, and with tramps who were looking for a billet. It was her practice to arrive at A&E at about 2am, where she would have a cup of tea and a chat with the staff on duty, before setting off on her rounds again. We assumed that there was a problem on one of the wards when she failed to appear one night. Early staff, arriving just after dawn, discovered what had befallen her.

The previous day, the hospital had received a delivery of coke. This was fed to the boiler room down a hatch at the side of the hospital. Darkness falls early in winter time, and nobody noticed that the hatch had not been replaced. During her night patrol, this unfortunate lady fell into the open hatch where she was trapped by her chest and could not extricate herself. Her injuries necessitated a long period away from work.

The Pathology Department was a separate building on the hospital site, just across from the ambulance entrance to the Accident and Emergency Department. Medical staff would often certify death at the entrance, so that the ambulance could continue towards the mortuary.

It was a beautiful summer evening when we heard the squeal of breaks as a car pulled up in the ambulance entrance. A young man ran in and shouted: 'It's my girlfriend!' I dashed to an open top sports car and found a blond, grey-faced young woman, with big pupils that did not react to light at all. Inspection of the back of the eye confirmed death, but I could find no injury.

There had been a minor collision, and without a seat belt, she had been thrown forward onto the walnut dashboard, which had a protruding ridge. (At the time, seatbelts were not compulsory, and cars were not fitted with them.) I wrote a short note to the Pathologist asking to be informed of the date and time of the autopsy. The configuration of the dashboard was explained to the Pathologist, and it was found that this young woman had died because her larynx had fractured on the protruding wooden ridge. A seat belt would have saved her, as there were no other injuries.

The motorway served by the hospital was a busy one, even then. It was Monday morning and a car was making the journey North. Approaching from the opposite direction at high speed was a second car, which crossed the central reservation and hit the North-bound vehicle head on. I certified the death of the North-bound driver in the back of the ambulance, noting that the deceased had a very wide face, probably unnaturally so, but there was no bleeding or other evidence of trauma. There were no other injuries.

The Pathologist began his examination with the head, and when the scalp was retracted, various-sized pieces of skull detached readily from the skull base. The remainder were removed, and the surface of the brain was revealed. The pathologist placed his fingers on the curved upper surface of the cerebral hemispheres. 'There is something extremely odd here, I can feel a very hard structure under my fingers.' He gently removed both cerebral hemispheres away from the brain stem and cerebellum. Right in the centre of the skull was the upper cervical spine, which had been hammered up through the skull base on impact.

At the time, the central reservation of a motorway was a space with no solid barrier to separate traffic moving in opposite directions.

The young man was tall, dark-haired and looked anxious. As he sat down, he said: 'I feel ill, and I am short of breath.' His temperature was normal. On examination, there were crackles at the bases of the lungs, suggesting the presence of fluid, but no dullness on percussion. A wheelchair and porter were summoned to get him to X-ray for a chest examination.

The resulting image alarmed me. It showed a much-enlarged heart shadow and short fine lines at the edge of the lung bases, consistent with heart failure. Urgent admission to a medical ward was arranged, and later that day he died.

Worries plagued me that I might have missed an abnormality in the heart valves, or perhaps a congenital defect. A brush with the Coroner was not to be desired.

At autopsy, both lungs were overloaded with fluid and could be squeezed out like bath sponges by the Pathologist. On slicing them, there was no sign of infection. To my relief, the heart valves were normal and there were no holes in the septum dividing the right and left sides of the heart. However, the heart muscle showed yellowish-white streaks, consistent with infection – with Coxsackie B, a virus that attacks heart muscle. Nothing could have been done for him at that time.

We saw little of the consultant physicians or surgeons at the hospital. From time to time, their registrars would be contacted about patients who, in our opinion, required admission. With one exception, they were helpful, and acknowledged that with the time and facilities at our disposal, we could not be expected to always get the diagnosis correct. The exception was Mr P, a surgical registrar who was usually scathing, and totally uncooperative.

It was ten at night and the town and environs were in darkness. A young woman was complaining of vomiting and right-sided abdominal pain at the level of her navel. Her periods were normal and she thought that something she had eaten had disagreed with her. The vomiting had not subsided.

There was no tenderness at the usual site of an inflamed appendix, but that structure is not always in the usual place. Gall bladder disease was unlikely, therefore further assessment and investigation were required. On balance, I considered the cause more likely to be surgical than medical. One thing was certain: she could not be sent home. Admittance was mandatory.

It was with a sinking feeling that I realised Mr L was the consultant surgeon taking emergencies, and I was going to have to deal with Mr P. As usual, he was sarcastic and uncooperative, scathing about my lack of knowledge and experience. Finally, he admitted that the patient could not be sent away and agreed to admit her.

When the department was quiet, I reflected on the incident and decided that enough was enough. Writing paper and envelope were assembled and I wrote to Mr L about the problems everyone at A&E was having with Mr P, I was no exception. The other registrars were cognisant of the difficulties of diagnosis in our department and accepted that we could not always get the diagnosis correct, but recognised that we were acting in the best interest of our patients.

The next evening at 5pm, I entered the Department to be told that Mr L was waiting for me in the Doctor's Office. I knew that a large slice of humble pie was going to be eaten and I mentally prepared an abject apology for wasting one of his surgical beds for a case which time had revealed to be medical.

As I opened the door of the office, my mouth opened to begin my prepared speech. Mr L made a movement with his hand to indicate that I was to be silent.

'Dr Percy, I have come to say thank you. That young patient you insisted on having admitted owes you her life. She had a ruptured ectopic pregnancy.' 'She cannot have. I asked specifically.' 'I know you did. I have read all your comments, but that is what it was.'

I learned later, through the grapevine, that when the abdomen was opened in theatre and found to be blood-filled, Mr L said to Mr P, 'This is your mess. Get yourself out of it.' then went and sat in a corner of the operating theatre. No trouble with Mr P after that.

The leg entered the department first in a bucket, followed by a young woman on a trolley with her crash helmet beside her. She had been knocked off her moped and sustained a traumatic amputation below the knee. There was virtually no bleeding, as the vessels had gone into spasm. She was conscious and was able to answer all questions sensibly.

No other injuries were detected.

A drip was set up and blood taken for blood chemistry and cross-matching. The orthopaedic registrar was informed at home. 'Is your department busy?' It was just after midnight and unusually quiet. I offered to admit her to the ward and carry out the necessary observations every quarter hour. During the remainder of the night, we chatted together at intervals, and she remained in good spirits, considering what had occurred.

At 8am the orthopaedic registrar arrived, and arrangements were made for her to go into the operating theatre to have the stump fashioned to take a prosthesis. I went off to bed, but returned to see her just before my duty began the following night.

She had no memory of the accident, her time in A&E or the events of the preceding night – perhaps a blessing.

During the night, the Sister in charge hailed from New Zealand, with much Maori blood in her veins. She was a valuable source of information and support. Once a wound had been properly assessed, she was quite prepared to get on and get it closed, freeing the one doctor on duty to attend to someone else.

Patients who arrived by ambulance needed undressing and clothing in a cotton hospital gown before examination, and between us, we had a system for such events. With the patient lying on their back on a trolley, Sister would deal with below the waist and I would manage the garments above that point. The patient was a man in his early twenties who had managed to turn his car over. This was explained in some detail as we went about our 'undressing the patient' routine. Sister tackled socks and shoes, while I undid the jacket and shirt buttons, and removed a tie. The next task was to slide garments out from beneath the patient and Mr K was asked to raise his bottom slightly off the trolley to enable this to be achieved.

As soon as his bottom began to rise, a hand flew immediately to the back of his neck. A cervical-supporting collar was placed around it. In this fashion, he went off to X-ray; no other injuries had been detected. The resulting images of his cervical spine were placed on light boxes in the medical staff room and showed a very serious injury with bone displacement. At that time the orthopaedic registrar was a tetchy South African and he had to be informed of the findings. It was 3:15am and he was at home.

Switchboard finally got him to answer the telephone. I stated who I was and at which hospital. I then gave the diagnosis I had made on the image of the patient's neck and added that movement and sensation at present were normal. 'Are you aware what time it is? You expect me to believe you on these images! I suppose you expect me to come and see the patient?' 'Yes, Mr S.' The telephone was crashed down.

Thirty minutes later, I was washing out a stomach behind a curtain. The ambulance door of the A&E unit was flung open and footsteps stomped down towards the medical staff room. The sliding door was propelled open with force and he must have entered. I was still busy behind the curtain with the stomach pump routine. The medical staff room was silent, and then I heard two words: 'Bloody Hell!'

Quiet footsteps approached the curtain behind which I was working, and Mr S entered. 'I need to get the car driver to theatre and insert tongs into his skull to start the reduction of that neck; perhaps you could assist if you are free. I will let you know when the anaesthetist is available.'

Later that week I was doing the night round on the Orthopaedic Ward. There was the car driver, flat on his back, metal tongs on either side of his skull attached to cords which went around a pulley to weights that pulled the bony constituents of the neck back into the correct position. He remembered me from his admission.

'You know, Dr Percy, I did not want to come into hospital at all. I wanted to go home, but you managed to persuade me. What would have happened had I done so?' 'You do not want to know.' 'But I do, so tell me.'

'There would have been loss of movement and sensation from the neck down – all four limbs involved.'

Every patient was an opportunity to learn something new. If we as individuals were unsure of anything, patients would be referred to consultant outpatient clinics. Rarely, a consultant could be contacted by telephone.

The balding elderly man was complaining of failing hearing in his ear. Neither accident nor emergency, but he had been registered as a patient, and I led the way to the cubicle with the ear and nose instruments to examine him. I expected to find nothing amiss, but a good light revealed a rounded mass behind the eardrum. Nothing like this had come my way before. The Ear Nose Throat consultant was surprised at my clinical findings and arranged for admission of the patient, later that day, to one of his beds in a neighbouring hospital.

After his operating list, he telephoned me with his findings. The mass I had seen was a large benign tumour which extended down towards the brain stem. He removed all that he could see and then realised that there was a similar tumour, of smaller size, on the opposite side of the head. That too was removed, but as an ENT surgeon he was uneasy about being close to vital areas of the brain.

Patients with eye injuries present quickly because of the intensity of the pain. 'Can you help me please?' The speaker was a tall man who had been carrying a small child on his shoulders. During the ride, the hand of the child had strayed from around Grandpa's neck and flicked in front of his face. A small, curved fingernail had scraped across the front of his eye and he was in agony. Once lying on the examination couch, local anaesthetic drops were instilled into the eye to aid examination and abolish pain for a while. The eye was red and angry. Use of a dye to highlight corneal damage showed a long scratch and then an ulcer. Local anaesthetic drops and an eye pad were required for some time until the healing process was complete.

Similar tactics were used with a little girl who had been playing in a sandpit when another child started flinging the sand around. She arrived screaming in the arms of her mother, both eyes screwed up. Quietness and firmness are necessary in such circumstances, and mother and daughter were told that we were going to the special eye room. Once there, while she was still in her mother's arms, I told her that my name was Doctor Percy and that I would help her, but she needed to lie down on the couch. Mother would be there to hold her hand, and would not leave her. She quietened and lay down with her mother on the right side of the couch. The cubicle wall was on her left, and I was at the head of the couch.

'The sand can be taken from your eyes without hurting them. To do that, special drops need to be dropped into your eyes. They sting at first a little, and then the pain will go, I promise you.'

Mother and daughter considered this, and I then had permission to put a drop into each eye. 'Tell me when they stop hurting.' It did not take long, and she was able to open both eyes and as much sand as possible could be washed out on each side. Both eyes were than protected with pads until the local anaesthetic wore off. A further treatment was necessary the following day, until every sand grain was removed. There was no problem in getting the cooperation of the child on that occasion.

Nursing Night Duty was divided between Sister M and Staff Nurse K, working alternate weeks. I could not understand why Staff Nurse was not a Sister as she had years of experience and was a hard worker. Day staff informed me that she had never shown any interest in being upgraded.

As my period of duty in the unit lengthened, I finally plucked up the courage one early morning when things were quiet to ask her why she remained a Staff Nurse. The answer was money. She was at the top of the Staff Nurse salary scale. An appointment as a Sister would involve an initial drop in salary and she could not afford it. Like Night Sister, she had no family in this country. She had to manage on her own.

A little younger than Sister M, she had brown permed hair with a tendency to be slightly frizzy, and bright blue eyes with a fresh complexion. Sister strode, Staff Nurse bustled. Sister could instil instant respect with a look that would freeze molten lava, Staff Nurse was verbally abused by a number of patients, some of them quite sober, because of her nationality. She was German.

On one of our nights on duty together, she was particularly chirpy, and confided over coffee that she had just signed the papers to buy a small terraced house. A structural survey had shown it to be sound, but the current appearance of the internal walls was definitely not to her taste. It would take time before she could save up for the decorator after the expense of the purchase.

'Do you intend to paint the walls or use wallpaper?' 'I doubt the walls would be good enough for just paint, that is why I need a decorator.'

'I can hang wallpaper; why don't we tackle this together?'

It was agreed that we would spend a period of time at the new house each day, before beginning a night shift, initially stripping off the old paper. Staff Nurse then sanded down and repainted while I worked days. By my next week of nights, the new wallpaper had been selected for the main bedroom and paperhanging began. It is much easier with two people and we were both pleased with the result.

By late spring, the refurbishment was well underway, but the new householder was not right. She looked tired, with dark circles under her eyes, and I was concerned. She assured me that there was no problem with her health, but that she had great difficulty sleeping on her nights off duty at this time of year.

As she began to drop off to sleep, and in her sleep, if she managed it, she could hear again the drone of the RAF Lancasters coming to bomb Berlin, where her family lived. They must have been very well connected, because Field Marshal Keitel was a neighbour, and as a child she played in the garden with the Keitel children.

There must have been quite a life story behind those bright blue eyes.

The hospital was fortunate in the calibre of surrounding GP practices. Referrals from them were invariably necessary. There was nobody like Dr W at the Borders Hospital, who was notorious for his diagnoses and treatment of his patients. Not all patients, however, would avail themselves of a general practitioner's knowledge. During the day, reception staff would redirect those attending Accident and Emergency with a rash, a toothache or a cough to the appropriate GP or dentist. At night there were no receptionists on duty, and a patient who woke at 3am with a sore throat got through the safety curtain. The antibiotic stock of the unit went down. The card index was always clearly marked: 'Should have seen GP in the morning.'

From time to time the medical staff were reminded that patients who were neither Accident nor Emergency were not our concern, and should be directed elsewhere – not always easy. Some patients returned with the same kind of complaint, having received prompt attention at the hospital on a prior occasion, and so repeated the process. A second attendance card was marked: 'Should see GP next time.'

It was late evening when the patient arrived. The receptionists had gone home. She complained of a sore throat and was told she should see her GP. 'But I have seen my GP and he gave me a prescription for these pills. I took two of them twenty minutes ago, but my throat is still sore.' 'You have not given enough time for the antibiotic prescribed to work. It has probably not entered your bloodstream yet.'

'Well, my throat still hurts, and my family want something else done.'

'If your GP has already begun treatment, it would be rude to interfere with his treatment, which is an appropriate antibiotic.'

'But my family want something done . . .'

I decided to telephone the GP and put him in the picture. The first dose of antibiotic was swallowed twenty-to-thirty minutes ago, and as yet, no miracle had occurred. He laughed down the telephone and said that as there was so much family anxiety, he would come to the hospital and see the patient again.

We met when he arrived. I offered to contact the Medical Registrar on his behalf if he had any anxieties about the patient, but after re-examining her, he was happy for the family to take her home and wait for the antibiotics to take effect.

When I arrived the following evening to begin work, the Consultant in charge was waiting for me. 'We need to talk about the lady with the sore throat whom you saw twenty-four hours ago.'

'I realise that we are not to function as an alternative GP service; we are for accidents and emergencies. She had already seen her GP, but expected the antibiotic to work almost instantly. The GP came in and saw her here. He was happy for her to go home. I did offer to contact the Medical Registrar on his behalf should he wish it, but he considered it unnecessary. I did try to do the best for the patient and the GP. On what grounds has a complaint been made?'

'Very simple. The patient is dead, possibly from meningitis spread from her infected throat. Fortunately for the hospital your notes are both legible and full. Try to attend the autopsy. No one has done anything wrong; it is just most unfortunate.'

It had been a hectic Saturday with multiple walking patients and the stretcher bays constantly full. A long anaesthetic session was necessary in our theatre for fracture and dislocation manipulation and the drainage of pus. The second on call had been summoned to help and had now left. The workload was now mine alone until day staff arrived to begin at 9am.

The ambulance klaxon could be heard as it approached the hospital, and grew ever-louder as the vehicle drove down the side entrance to approach our department. The noise of the bell ceased and was replaced by the screams of a child. An ambulance man ran towards me. 'A child has been scalded.'

He went to Reception to give details. I moved towards the screaming child and her distraught parents. The clothing had been removed and the bright pink, scalded flesh with large blisters filling with fluid extended over the back and upper chest. There was a little blistering on the neck and lower face.

The Regional Burns Unit did not accept cases from A&E, only from wards. The Paediatric wards were in a neighbouring hospital, closer to the centre of town. I telephoned the Senior House Officer in Paediatrics and gave him details of the extent and severity of the damage.

Instructions were received on the type of dressing to be applied before the child was transferred. Good pain relief would be necessary before any treatment was attempted. I wrote up the prescription for the analgesia, remembering the simple system 1 minim per year of age. The drug was administered by injection into one of the areas of undamaged skin by the nursing staff. Dressings could be applied when the drug began to take effect.

It took quite some time for an ambulance to become available to transfer child and parents to the other hospital, but the parents were happy to wait now that their daughter was comfortable. The department was still heaving.

Some two to three hours later the telephone rang in the medical staff room. It was the Paediatric SHO calling about the scalded child. 'One final point, Dr Percy: did you write up the prescription for the analgesia?' 'Yes, one minim per year of age.' 'One minim per year of age, but she is not yet one year old.'

There is a sickening feeling in the pit of the stomach that accompanies the realisation of a horrendous mistake. I had prescribed an overdose. Visions of the Coroner and the National Press loomed in my mind, coupled with the parents' devastation.

'She is under our care and we will watch her. I will ring you in the morning before you go off duty.'

When not attending to patients that night, I paced the floor. Visions of the Coroner and the National Press had been joined by the General Medical Council and being struck off the Medical Register.

It was 7:50am when the telephone rang.

'Good morning Dr Percy. I have a message for you from the parents of the scalded child. They are delighted with the treatment you gave to their daughter. She was in agony, and thanks to you, she has slept all night. We have said nothing. So, to bed, Doctor, and stop worrying. All is well!'

A good sense of smell can be a mixed blessing for a doctor. It confers the ability to detect an impending diabetic coma by the chemicals in the breath of the patient and the certain knowledge that a bowel containing altered blood has just emptied. The smell is unmistakable.

A bright little girl of four years of age was brought in by her mother because of a peculiar smell. It appeared to arise from the face of the child, and the mother thought that she may have a sinus infection. Dr T shook his head. 'The sinuses have not formed at this age.' He knelt down to the level of the child's face and asked quietly: 'What did you push up?'

'A leaf.'

A good light directed up the nostril showed the lower edge of a curled piece of foliage which was retrieved with fine tweezers. It was followed by a trickle of revolting gunk. The leaf was the first botanical specimen some of us had encountered. More usually, it was a ball bearing, paper, or a piece of toy.

Dr H was a forthright anaesthetist from South Africa. The final case, after the fractures and dislocations had been dealt with, was a large abscess to be drained. I had on a mackintosh apron over my white coat. The patient was anaesthetised on the theatre table – we had no anaesthetic room. I waited by the trolley of instruments for a nod from Dr H to let me know I could begin.

Once seen, I approached with my trolley, prepared the skin and arranged the surgical drapes. Then the scalpel was directed down into the most inflamed area. Pus ejected at force directly towards my face and head. Spectacles were quickly removed by Staff Nurse; a mask shielded my lower face, but my brow and the hair above were drenched.

Once the cavity of the drained abscess had been packed with ribbon gauze and the patient was returning to consciousness, Dr H took charge. 'You need to go and shampoo your hair. Staff Nurse will let you out of the fire escape door so that you contaminate as little as possible of this department. I will explain to Mr B where you have gone and why. Quite frankly, Dr Percy, at present, you stink.'

Working in a busy department had given me experience in reducing various fractures and dislocated joints in the limbs. One fracture we knew always to notify a consultant about, was a fracture just above the elbow in a child. The brachial artery, the blood supply to the hand and forearm, lies just anterior to the bone above the elbow and was the most important structure to protect. If the artery went into spasm or was damaged, the child could be left with a deformity. If the arm was held straight by the child, it was never to be bent and placed in a sling, but left as it was. The most important examination was to feel for the pulse at the wrist and document whether or not it was present. If already absent, speedy consultant attention was required. If present, quarter hourly observations were required, and a referral made.

In order to gain more experience in managing serious trauma than I had already acquired, the 'Situations Vacant' section of The Lancet and the British Medical Journal were studied. I applied for a post at a busy Midlands hospital and was successful at interview. It meant moving North, which would be a change. Leaving the Armistice was a wrench. I had learned a great deal, and would look back on my time there with great affection and gratitude.

The Midlands Centre

My new appointment was still at Senior House Officer level. I joined one of three teams of medical staff providing twenty-four-hour trauma cover. Each team was led by two consultant surgeons, supported by a Senior Registrar, a Registrar and three SHO's. I was to be one of the latter.

The hospital was quite separate from other buildings and away from the city centre. The ground floor was largely occupied by a standard Accident and Emergency Unit, similar to those at which I had previously worked. The new feature for me was a Major Injuries Unit which could cope with multiple trauma cases. There were sufficient operating theatres for both consultants and the Senior Registrar to be operating at the same time. The remaining junior staff then maintained the service on the ground floor.

There was a busy x-ray department and the consultant radiologist visited twice weekly to review all images since his previous visit, in case an injury had been missed. As before, the skull was imaged in three planes: from the side, back and front. What was going on inside the skull had to be deduced by clinical examination and meticulous monitoring of the vital signs.

Everyone was intrigued when one of the consultants bought a piece of equipment to assist in assessing the contents of the skull. He explained to us that when the device was plugged into an electricity socket, one of the two small contact discs would emit a beam of very high-pitched sound, inaudible to the human ear. If the contact discs were placed on either side of the head, a beam of sound would go through the skull and across the brain; the midline structures of the brain would cause an upward spike on the small screen of the device, because they were of a different nature to the brain itself. The sound beam would then continue across the brain on the other side of the midline and be reflected back from the inner table of the skull.

It was pointed out to us that using the device would enable bleeding on one side of the head to be detected, because the midline structures would have moved towards the skull on the opposite side. It would then be possible to drill down towards the haemorrhage and release the blood. Unfortunately, bleeding on both sides would still be a problem. This was an introduction to the medical use of ultrasound.

Inevitably, there were periods of quiet, which junior staff used for study, sitting on the examination couches of the Outpatient area. One did need to be wary. One of the consultants delighted in distending rubber gloves with water and hanging them from the curtain rails around the examination couches. He would then throw a dart, which was a small plastic syringe with needle attached, at the rubber glove, and attempt to shower the junior staff!

Renown in surgery may not be accompanied by common sense. Mr H had walked through the quiet Outpatient department towards the car park. He reappeared quite quickly and walked towards the telephone on the centre desk. Switchboard was asked to connect him to his home.

'My dear, I will be late, and have no idea when I will arrive. My car has been stolen and I need to inform the police, which I will do as soon as I have finished speaking to you. Goodness knows how long it will all take.'

There was a period of silence as Mrs H spoke to her spouse. When she had finished, the receiver was replaced, and he turned towards me, looking sheepish.

'My wife informs me that my car has not been stolen. I took it to the garage this morning for a service and should have collected it before five. Too late now; I must get a taxi, and collect it tomorrow.'

One of my responsibilities was to inject a steroid into stiff joints to aid mobilisation. This was done in an operating theatre with full sterile procedure to prevent infection occurring. Rumour had it that there had been an incident in the fairly recent past. This was odd, because one of the consultants was operating in normal indoor clothes under a surgical gown. The explanation advanced by Senior Registrar was that he had just returned to work after a heart attack. This made no sense, as he surely changed into pyjamas for bed. If I was using full sterile procedure to insert a sterile needle into a joint, he was working with an open wound – the risk was surely higher?

The vast majority of our patients were adults. I was still wary of anything to do with children, but late one autumn afternoon, we received a small girl who had been hit by a car. There was significant damage to her face, including a broken jaw. She was to go to the operating theatre for surgery to stabilise the fractures. A drip of cross-matched blood was in place, and I was monitoring both child and drip. A consultant came over and perused the child, charts and drip. 'The drip is too rapid, Dr Percy. This is a child. We do not want her to go into heart failure because of fluid overload.' He adjusted the rate of flow and then left for the operating theatre to prepare for the child.

Next morning, I asked the Senior Registrar about the little girl and was told that she had died. This was a shock. Some days later, he sought me out to discuss events. The inquiry into the death of the child had concluded that the underlying cause was blood loss. Why had I set the drip at such a low rate? I explained that the speed of the drip had been set by a consultant who had talked about the danger of heart failure with a drip that, in his opinion, was too rapid.

'And you saw him slow the speed of the drip?'

'Yes. I had to abide by what he had set. I take no responsibility for under transfusion. I was overruled.'

Sometime later, my future career came under discussion. Trauma perhaps was not a suitable choice for a female doctor. 'It has been noticed that you have an aptitude for interpretation of x-ray images. Have you considered training in Radiology?'

The answer was no, but I thought about my postgraduate experience of Medicine. There was certainly an unspoken antagonism towards women in Surgery, particularly trauma and orthopaedics. I did enjoy the challenge of interpreting x-ray images, which were shadows cast by anatomical structures. I had loved Anatomy as a student. Radiology was applied Anatomy. I made a decision – I would go towards the shadows.

Epilogue

It has been our practice to meet every five years in the city where we trained during a weekend in September. We gather on Friday, and there is an evening buffet meal. Organised activity may take place on Saturday afternoon, and the evening is marked by a black-tie dinner with a guest speaker. Each meal begins with us standing in silence to remember our dead. The numbers grow with the passing of the years.

Some colleagues never come, others are nearly always there. They come from Australia, Canada, the USA, Finland and an island in the Indian Ocean. After the speeches, frequently given by those who helped to train us, there is an opportunity to mingle and chat, often with those we have not seen for many years.

The love birds J and J came to the forty-fifth reunion. They had married shortly after graduation, become general practitioners and raised a family. The wife had struck up a conversation about plants with me, a subject in which we both shared an interest. Her husband later joined us, and she drifted away to speak to someone else.

As he and I talked quietly, his face hardened.

'There is Alec South, the bastard, and still no hint of an apology.'

'Maybe', I said, 'he has nothing to apologise for.'

'Don't you take that line with me, Anona, I am absolutely certain that he was responsible for all those pranks played on us.'

'Why is that?'

'Look, there were eight of us in residence and J and I were in the same room. That leaves six individuals, some of whom were responsible for unscrewing that door handle. It could not be Pamela and it would not be you. It was one of those four men, and by far the most likely was Alec South. I know it was him.' He was indignant.

'Then you are wrong, because it was not.'

'Do you know who it was then?'

'Of course, I have always known, right from the beginning.'

'So, who was it then?'

'It was me.'

A look of stupefaction came over his face. A silence commenced, followed by his quiet remark.

'Still waters certainly do run deep.'

I smiled. 'You had me conveniently pigeonholed as a boring God-botherer. I am quite mischievous underneath!'

It was many years before I realised what was going on in my viva on surgical instruments, and why the Professor was so annoyed.

In steering me backwards across the room, he was manoeuvring me towards the instruments used in upper abdominal surgery: his field of expertise. There was, however, something about me that he did not know, something he had not considered in his plan. Like my father, I am left handed. My right hand made no move towards the instruments of his choice, but my left descended into the orthopaedic steel.

What compounded his problem was that I had described a new surgical procedure in Paediatric Orthopaedics, a niche subject. The Professor may have had no exposure to Orthopaedics since his student days, and had no way of knowing if what I was saying was correct. It may have been the Paediatric equivalent of 'Mary had a Little Lamb.' He was out of his depth – and he was the examiner. No wonder he was furious. That was, however, no excuse for what followed.

Richard Davies (from the Rhondda) became a consultant anaesthetist, providing care to patients undergoing cardiothoracic surgery in the city of our training.

David Ladds became a consultant anaesthetist in a city with a magnificent cathedral.

Both men died in the same year with non-malignant chest problems.

Neville Playfair did not complete his training. Last known fish farming off the west coast of Scotland.

Dr B, demonstrator in Anatomy, became Professor of Surgery at a neighbouring centre with a special interest in breast cancer. Now deceased.

Lynne Dye – Professor of Paediatric Cancer in San Francisco.

Patience Rawlings – GP in London.

Mary Duckworth —- Family Planning?

2017 marks fifty years since our graduation and much has changed in Medicine, in the city, and in the way we look. This is a record of how it was, when we were the Golden Girls and Guys of 1967.